Ashwagandha
(*Withania somnifera*)
Activities and
Applications of the
Versatile Ayurvedic Herb

Saligrama C. Subbarao
Lakshmi Subbarao
Bruce Ferguson

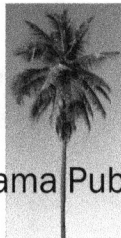

Saligrama Publishing

Published by Saligrama Publishing.

Contact the primary author at saligrama_subbarao@yahoo.com

ISBN 978-0-9843812-3-4

Printed in the United States of America

The information presented in this book is intended for educational purposes only, not as medical advice. The publisher and authors disclaim all responsibility for any liability, loss or risk associated with the use of the information presented in this book.

I warmly dedicate this book to

My late younger brother Athri Sharma, a kind, honest and simple person

-SCS

Acknowledgments

From *Saligrama Subbarao:*

At the outset, I want to thank all of the scientists who have published on Ashwagandha. Without their publications, this book could not have been written.

I would like to thank my wife Mythili, son Kartik and daughter Lakshmi for their interest, support and encouragement. I want to thank my sisters Vedavathi Govindaraju, Manjula Laxminarasimhiah, Shambhavi Vijayasarathy and my late brother Athri Sharma's wife Jayashree for their encouragement. I would like to thank my nephew Meghanath Laxminarasimhiah for supervising the typing of this work in India.

I want to thank my friends Mahinder Chopra and his wife Swaran Chopra for their encouragement. I would like to thank my friends Dr. Ramachandra Bhat, R. Shivashankar and Parthasarathy for their encouragement. My thanks to Dr. Robert Abel, whose holistic attitude in the treatment of patients is an inspiratio. My coauthors Lakshmi Subbarao and Bruce Ferguson deserve special thanks. Their rich and varied experience were invaluable to the preparation of this book.

Finally, I would like to thank Kartik Subbarao, Chief Editor of Saligrama Publishing. He meticulously read numerous drafts of the manuscript and thoroughly edited them. He also designed the organization and layout of the book. His patient and tireless efforts made the completion of this book possible.

Preface

Ashwagandha (Withania somnifera) is a well-known medicinal plant in Ayurveda, the traditional system of Indian medicine. The major Ayurvedic texts such as Charaka Samhita (about 1000 BC), Sushruta Samhita (1000-500 BC) and Ashtanga Hridaya (500-600 AD) have described various therapeutic uses of Ashwagandha. In India, Ashwagandha has been used for thousands of years to maintain good health as well as to prevent or cure a number of psychological and physical disorders. Nowadays, Ashwagandha is known all over the world. Over the last few decades, a considerable amount of work has been done to scientifically verify the therapeutic efficacy of Ashwagandha as mentioned in Ayurveda texts. Extensive in vitro and in vivo studies as well as limited clinical studies indicate beneficial effects for various disorders.

This book provides in one place a summary of results published in various journals. Its intent is to serve as an accessible reference and guide for formulators, R&D professionals, biomedical researchers and medical practitioners.

Table of Contents

1 – Introduction

1.1 – General

Ashwagandha is one of the most highly valued medicinal plants. It has been extensively used in Ayurveda, the traditional Indian system of medicine, for more than 3000 years to preserve good health and treat a wide variety of physical and psychological disorders. In Ayurveda, Ashwagandha is well known as a rasayana. Rasayanas enhance vitality, rejuvenate body tissues, and mitigate the ill effects of aging. Ashwagandha belongs to a subgroup of rasayanas known as medhya rasayanas, which are specific to the brain and nervous system. These have been traditionally used to reduce cognitive decline as well as to preserve and enhance cognitive functions.

Ashwagandha has an official status as an adaptogen in the Indian Herbal Pharmacopoeia[1]. It is mentioned in the World Health Organization (WHO) monographs on the most important medicinal plants. It has been included in the list of top 32 prime concerned medicinal plants by the National Medical Plant Board of India[2].

Ashwagandha is a Sanskrit word that literally means "scent of a horse". This name was probably used because the fresh roots of the plant smell like a sweaty horse. The plant also has the reputation of imparting the strength and vitality of a stallion to the user[3]. The scientific name for Ashwagandha is Withania somnifera. In Latin, somnifera means "sleep-inducing", indicating the sleep-enhancing property of the plant[4]. Ashwagandha is also known as winter cherry and Indian ginseng[5].

During the last few decades, the popularity of Ashwagandha has spread all over the world, including Europe and the US. It has made its way into a large number of health food stores. It has also attracted the attention of scientists and health professionals. Scientific investigations are progressing in many parts of the world to test the validity of the varied Ayurvedic applications of Ashwagandha and also to explore new benefits.

1.2 – Ashwagandha in Classic Ayurvedic Literature

Ashwagandha is prominent in the materia medica of Ayurveda. It is described in major Ayurvedic texts such as Charaka Samhita[6], Sushruta Samhita[7] and Ashtanga Hridaya[8] (major triad), where it is acclaimed as a versatile medicinal plant. Recently, reviews of Ashwagandha based on Ayurvedic Samhitas and Nighantus have been published[9,10].

1.3 – Ayurvedic Pharmacological Properties of Ashwagandha

Ayurvedic pharmacological properties of Ashwagandha are presented below[11,12]:

- Rasa: Madhura, Kashaya, Tikta
- Guna: Laghu, Snigdha
- Veerya: Ushna
- Vipaka: Madhura

1.4 – Synonyms in Sanskrit

Ashwagandha is known by a number of other names in Sanskrit, including Asgandha, Balya, Haya, Kustagandhin, Vajikari, Varahakarni, Vagigandha, Varda, Vatahara, and Vrsha[11,12].

1.5 – Ayurvedic Uses of Ashwagandha

Ashwagandha is used in Ayurveda to maintain good health as well as to prevent, cure or control a wide variety of disorders. The therapeutic uses include treatment of skin disorders (kusta), fever (jwara), pulmonary tuberculosis (rajayakshama), abdominal disorders (udara roga), asthma (shwast), cough (kasa), neurological disorders (vatavyadhi), gout (vatarakta), emaciation (karshya roga), inflammation (kaphajsopha), wounds (vrana), insanity (unmada), cardiac disorders (hridroga), vaginal disorders (yonivyapada), fertility disorders (nandhyavata), epilepsy (apasmara), diabetes (pramehapidika), tumors (arubda) and a host of other disorders[12,13].

1.6 – Description, Habitat and Cultivation

Withania somnifera is a short, erect shrub with a main stem from which branches extend radially. The stem and branches are covered with dense wool-like hairs. The plant grows to a height of 150 cm. It is covered by ovate green leaves and bears green/yellow flowers. The plant produces small, round, red berry-like fruits. The seeds are yellow and kidney-shaped. The roots are stout, fleshy, whitish-brown and aromatic.

Withania somnifera is widely distributed across the globe. It is found throughout the drier parts of India, Baluchistan, Afghanistan, Pakistan, Bangladesh, Nepal and Sri Lanka, as well as in different parts of Australia, Africa and America. In India, Ashwagandha is cultivated in Madhya Pradesh, Gujarat, Maharashtra, Rajasthan, Haryana, Punjab, Karnataka and Uttar Pradesh. Ashwagandha grows well in areas receiving about 500–750 mm rainfall annually and at altitudes between 600–1200 m. Temperatures between 20–38 °C are suitable for its cultivation. It grows well in sandy loam or light red soil with pH 7.5–8 and good drainage. The crop is populated either by broadcast seeding or line sowing, the latter being preferred as it increases root production. Seeds are also germinated in nursery beds; subsequently, six-week-old seedlings are transplanted late in the rainy season around August–September. The plants start flowering and bearing fruits in February–March and the crop is ready for harvesting in April–May[14-17].

1.7 – Taxonomical classification

The taxonomical classification of Withania somnifera is presented below[4]:

- Kingdom: Plantae
- Subkingdom: Tracheobionta, Vascular plants
- Superdivision: Spermatophyta, Seed plants
- Division: Angiospermae
- Class: Dicotyledons
- Order: Tubiflorae
- Family: Solanaceae
- Genus: Withania
- Species: Somnifera Dunal

1.8 – Constituents

The chemistry of Withania somnifera has been extensively investigated during the last several decades. It is a rich reservoir of a diverse group of chemicals that have therapeutic potential. Most of its health benefits are attributed to the biochemical constituents known as withanolides. Withanolides are a group of naturally-occurring C28 steroidal lactones built on an ergostane frame structure. The withanolide skeleton is defined as 22-hydroxyergostan–26-oic acid–26,22-lactone.

There are many novel structural variants of withanolides with modifications to either the carbocyclic skeleton or side chain. In addition to withanolides, different classes of withanosides, glycowithanolides, sitoindosides, alkaloids, saponins, amino acids, flavonoids, phenolic compounds and others with therapeutic activity are present[18]. Iron, copper, nickel, manganese and zinc have also been found[19]. The structures of several compounds present in Withania somnifera are shown below (Table 1.1).

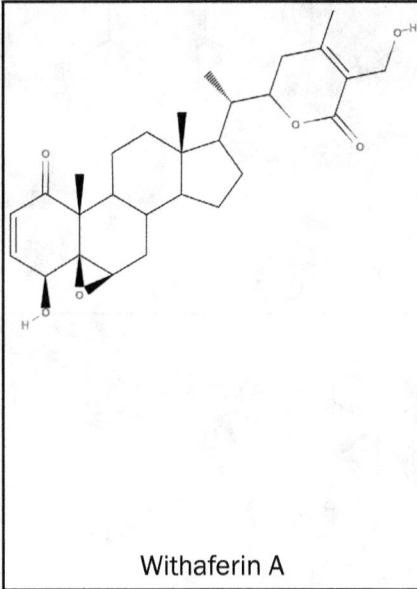

Withaferin A

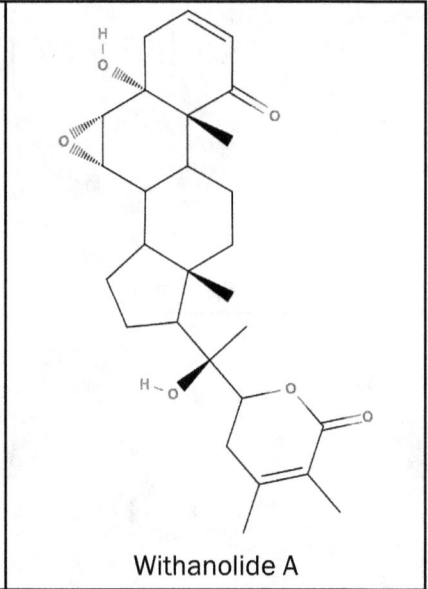

Withanolide A

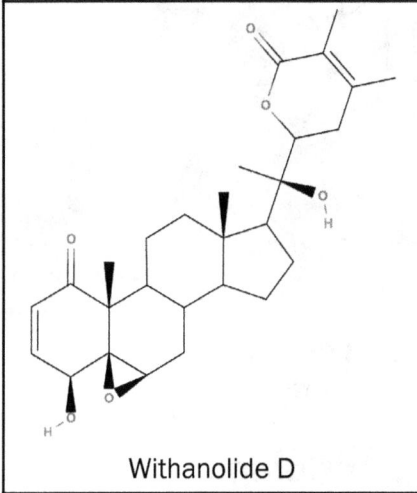

Withanolide D

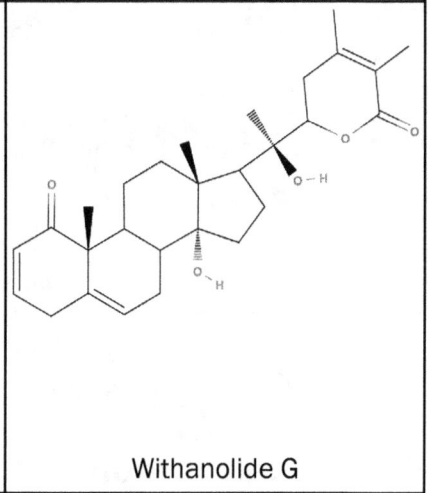

Withanolide G

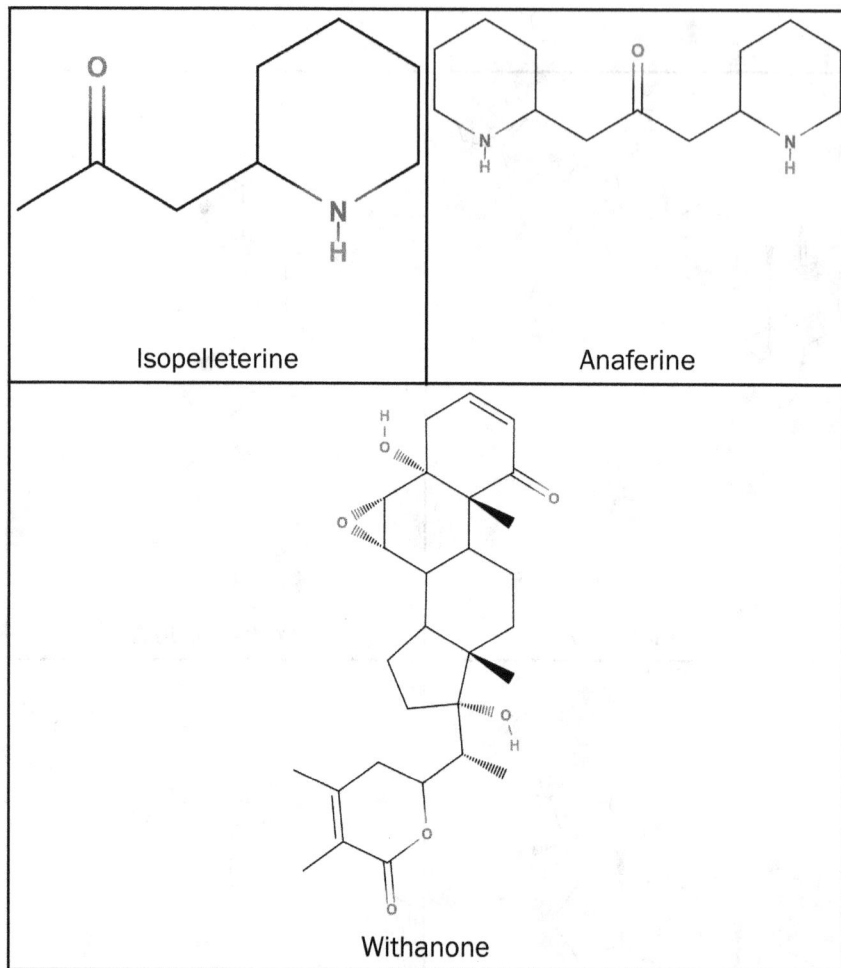

Isopelleterine

Anaferine

Withanone

Table 1.1: Structures of Selected Compounds Found in Withania Somnifera

1.9 – Quantitation of Major Components

High performance thin layer chromatography (HPTLC) and high performance liquid chromatography (HPLC) are commonly used in the quantitation of major components. HPTLC is an advanced form of conventional thin layer chromatography. Key features of HPTLC include the following[20]:

- simplicity, speed and cost-effectiveness

- minimum sample clean-up

- high sample throughput

- simultaneous processing of sample and standards
- minimum consumption of organic solvents and minimum waste production
- no interference from previous analyses
- reproducibility, accuracy, reliability and robustness

Reversed phase HPLC has become the standard technique for the analysis of Withania somnifera and its formulations. With proper optimization of the stationary phase, mobile phase, flow rate, temperature, etc., even structurally similar components can be separated.

A summary of results from select publications is presented in Table 1.2 (HPTLC) and Table 1.3 (HPLC).

Stationary Phase	Silica Gel 60 F_{254} pre-coated TLC plates		
Mobile Phase	Toluene:Ethyl acetate:Formic acid (5:5:1)		
Temperature	25 °C	Solvent Front Migration	90 mm
Relative Humidity	50%	Detection Scan	530 nm absorption-reflection mode
Validation Parameters		Withaferin A	Withanolide A
	Linearity Range (ng)	200–3200	200–3200
	r	0.999	0.9999
	LOD (ng)	120	160
	LOQ (ng)	800	800
	% Recovery	95.6–96.3	96.2–97.3
Reference	21		

Stationary Phase	Silica Gel G60 F_{254} HPTLC plates		
Mobile Phase	Chloroform:Methanol:Toluene:Formic acid (6.5:0.5:3.0:0.25 V/V)		
Solvent Front Migration	80 mm		
Detection Scan	530 nm absorption-reflection mode		
Validation Parameters		Withaferin A	Stigmasterol
	Linearity Range (ng)	100–600 ng	200–700 ng
	r^2	0.9960	0.9931
	LOD (ng/band)	23.82	10.05
	LOQ (mg/band)	72.18	30.46
	% Recovery	100.06–100.46	99.7–100.94
Precision (%RSD)	Repeatability	0.24–1.26	0.63–1.23
	Intermediate Precision	0.74–1.51	0.75–0.95
Reference	22		

Stationary Phase	Silica Gel 60 F_{254} coated on aluminum baked plates		
Mobile Phase	Toluene:ethyl acetate:Methanol:Formic acid (60:8:5:1)		
Temperature	28 °C **Solvent Front Migration** 80 mm		
Detection Scan	220 nm		
Validation Parameters		Withaferin A	Withanolide A
	Linearity Range (ng/band)	400–3200	400–3200
	r^2	0.999	0.999
	LOD (ng/band)	1.58	2.65
	LOQ (ng/band)	4.8	8.03
	% Recovery	98.13	99.16
Reference	23		

Stationary Phase	Silica Gel 60 F_{254} precoated on aluminum backed plates		
Mobile Phase	Chloroform:Methanol (8:2 V/V)		
Temperature	25 °C	Solvent Front Migration	8 cm
Relative Humidity	60%	Detection Scan	207 nm reflectance-absorbance mode
Validation Parameters		Withaferin A	Beta-Sitosterol-D-Glucoside
	Linearity Range (µg/ml)	0.5–5	5–500
	r^2	0.9991	0.9995
	LOD (ng/ml)	100	10
	LOQ (µg/ml)	300	30
	% Recovery	101.66–103.21	97.86–99.01
Reference	24		

Stationary Phase	Aluminum Backed Silica Gel 60 F_{254}
Mobile Phase	Toluene:Ethyl acetate:Formic acid (8:4:0.6 V/V/V)
Detection Scan	235 nm reflectance-absorbance mode
Validation Parameters		Withaferin A
	Linearity Range (ng/spot)	100–400
	r^2	0.999
	LOD (ng/spot)	30
	LOQ (mg/spot)	80
	% Recovery	98–102
Reference	25

Table 1.2: Summary of HPTLC Results

Column	Phenomenex Luna C18 (250 x 4.6 mm, 5 µm)		
Mobile Phase	A: Phosphate Buffer; B: Acetonitrile		
Elution (Gradient)	10 - 20% B in 12 min; 20 - 45% B in 6 min; 45 - 80% B in 7 min; 80% B for 3 min; 80 - 45% B in 7 min; 45 - 10% B in 5 min; 10% B for 5 min		
Compounds Analyzed	quercetin 3-O-robinobioside-7-O-glucoside quercetin 3-O-rutinoside-7-O-glucoside kaempferol 3-O-robinoside-7-O-glucoside		
Flow Rate	1.5 ml/min	Injection Volume	20 µl
Column Temperature	27 °C	Detection Wavelength	UV at 350 nm
Validation Parameters	Linearity Range: 10–550 µg/ml r^2: 0.9995–0.9996 LOD: 0.5 µg/ml LOQ: 1.5 µg/ml %RSD: 1.38–2.10 (intra-day), 1.22–1.58 (inter-day) % Recovery: 91–107		
Reference	26		

Column	Phenomenex Luna C18(2) (250 x 4.6 mm, 5 µm)		
Mobile Phase	A: Acetonitrile; B: Water		
Elution (Isocratic)	50% A : 50% B		
Compound Analyzed	Withaferin A		
Flow Rate	1 ml/min	Injection Volume	20 µl
Column Temperature	27 °C	Detection Wavelength	PDA at 225 nm
Validation Parameters	Linearity Range: 0.005%–0.02% r^2: 0.993 % Recovery: 94.4		
Reference	27		

Column	C18 (5 µm)
Mobile Phase	A: Methanol + 0.05% trimethylamine B: Water + 0.05% trimethylamine
Elution (Isocratic)	98% A : 2% B
Compound Analyzed	Withaferin A
Flow Rate	1 ml/min	Injection Volume	20 µl

Detecion Wavelength	UV at 227 nm
Validation Parameters	**Linearity Range:** 5–30 µg/ml **r²:** 0.999 **LOD:** 1.48 µg/ml **LOQ:** 4.48 µg/ml **%RSD:** 0.8 (intra-day), 0.76 (inter-day) **% Recovery:** 97.3
Reference	28

Column	Merck LiChrospher RP-18e (250 x 4 mm, 5 µm)
Mobile Phase	A: Acetonitrile; B: Water
Elution (Isocratic)	50% A : 50% B
Compound Analyzed	Withanolide A
Flow Rate	1 ml/min	Injection Volume	20 µl
Column Temperature	30 °C	Detection Wavelength	PDA at 240 nm

Validation Parameters	**Linearity Range:** 2–100 µg/ml **r²:** 0.999 **LOD:** 0.5 µg/ml **LOQ:** 2 µg/ml **% Recovery:** 97.5–100.75
Reference	29

Column	Nucleosil C18 (250 x 4.6 mm)		
Mobile Phase	A: Acetonitrile; B: Water		
Elution (isocratic)	60% A: 40% B	**Injection Volume**	4 µl
Flow Rate	1 ml/min	**Column Temperature**	35 °C
Detectors	DAD: 215 nm ELSD: evaporation temperature 45 °C; nitrogen pressure 4 bar		
Validation Parameters		Withaferin A	Withanolide A
	Linearity Range (µg/ml)	60–140	
	DAD r^2	0.9995	0.9996
	ELSD r^2	0.9921	0.9945
	DAD LOD (µg/ml)	2.29	2.07
	ELSD LOD (µg/ml)	9.33	7.77
	DAD LOQ (µg/ml)	6.95	6.27
	ELSD LOQ (µg/ml)	28.29	23.56
	DAD % Recovery	96.76	98.42
	ELSD % Recovery	96.96	98.81
Reference	30		

Column	Phenomenex Synergi MAX-RP 80 Å (150 x 4.6 mm, 4 µm)		
Mobile Phase	A: Water; B: 50% Methanol : 50% Ethanol		
Elution (gradient)	35 - 45% B in 25 min; 100% B for 5 min; 35% B for 10 min		
Flow Rate	1.0 ml/min	**Detection Wavelength**	PDA at 230 nm
Injection Volume	10 µl		
Validation Parameters		Withaferin A	Withanolide D
	Linearity Range (µg/ml)	1.6–400	
	r^2	0.9996	
	LOD (µg/ml)	0.26	0.23
	% Recovery	97.59	100
Reference	31		

Column	Merck LiChrospher (250 x 4.6 mm, 5 µm)		
Mobile Phase	A: Acetonitrile: B: Water		
Elution (isocratic)	45% A : 55% B		
Flow Rate	0.8 ml/min	Column Temperature	27 °C
Validation Parameters		Withaferin A	Withanolide A
	Linearity Range (µg/ml)	1-16	
	r^2	0.999	
	LOD (µg/ml)	0.13	0.27
	LOQ (µg/ml)	0.39	0.83
	% RSD	1.7	0.5
	% Recovery	95.98	97.1
Reference	32		

Column	Phenomenex Luna C18(2) (250 x 4.6 mm, 5 µm)	
Mobile Phase	A: Acetonitrile; B: Water	
Elution (isocratic)	60% A : 40% B	
Flow Rate	1 ml/min	Column Temperature	Ambient
Injection Volume	20 µl	Detection	UV at 230 nm
Validation Parameters	Linearity Range (µg/ml)	2-20
	r^2	0.999
	LOD (µg/ml)	0.05
	LOQ (µg/ml)	0.16
	% RSD	0.12–1.55 (intra-day) 0.04–1.73 (inter-day)
	% Recovery	99.43–100.64
Reference	33	

Table 1.3: Summary of HPLC Results

References

1   M. S. Premila. Ayurvedic Herbs: a clinical guide to the healing plants of traditional Indian medicine. The Haworth Press Inc, Binghamton, NY, 2006.

2   Pritika Singh, Rupam Guleri, Amrita Angurala, Kuldeep Kaur, Kulwinder Kaur, Sunil C. Kaul, Renu Wadhwa, and Pratap Kumar Patil. Addressing challenges to enhance the bioactives of Withania somnifera through organ, tissue, and cell culture based approaches. BioMed Research International, volume 2017, Article ID 3278494, 15 pages.

3   K. Chandrasekhar, Jyoti Kapoor, Sridhar Anishetty. A prospective, randomized double-blind, placebo-controlled study of safety and efficacy of a high concentration full-spectrum extract of ashwagandha root in reducing the stress and anxiety in adults. Indian Journal of Psychological Medicine (2012) 34 (3): 255- 262.

4   Chaurasia Pratibha, Bora Madhumati, Parihar Akarsh. Therapeutic properties and significance of different parts of Ashwagandha- a medicinal plant. International Journal of Pure & Applied Biosciences (2013) 1 (6): 94-101.

5   Shreesh Kumar Ojha and Dharamvir Singh Arya. Withania somnifera Dunal (Ashwagandha): A promising remedy for cardiovascular diseases. World journal of Medical Sciences (2009) 4 (2): 156-158.

6   Caraka Samhita (Text with english translation & critical exposition based on Cakrapani Duttas Ayurveda Dipika). By R. K. Sharma and Bhagwan Dash. Chowkhama Sanskrit Series Office, Varanasi, India.

7   Illustrated Susruta Samhita (Text, English translation, Notes, Appendeces and Index). Translator: K. R. Srikantha Murthy. Chaukhamba Orientalia, Varanasi, India.

8   Vagbhata's Astanga Hrdayam (Text, English translation, Notes, Appendix indices) Translated by: K. R. Srikantha Murthy. Chowkhamba Krishnadas Academy, Varanasi, India.

9   Satya Prakash Chaudhary. An Ayurvedic review of Ashwagandha from Samhitha and Nighatus. World Journal of Pharmaceutical Research (2015) 4 (10): 2736-2745.

10   Pratibha, Sudipta Kumar Rath. Medicinal uses of Ashwagandha (Indian Ginseng) - A historical review. International Journal of Science and Research Methodology (2017) 7 (1): 149-162.

11   Harish Kumar Singhal, Neetu, Amit Kataria and Jai Singh Yadav. A review on Ashwagandha (Withania somnifera (L) Dunal). Int J Ayu Pharm Chem (2014) 1(1): 142–157.

12   Dravyaguna Vijnana, 3rd edition. Gyanendra Pandey. Chowkhamba Krishnadas Academy. Varanasi, India, 2005.

13   Krutika J, Swagata Tavhare, Kalpesh Panara, Praveen Kumar A, Nishteswar Karra. Studies of Ashwagandha (Withania somnifera Dunal). International Journal of Pharmaceutical & Biological Archives (2016) 7 (1): 1-11.

14   Qamar Uddin, L. Samiulla, V. K. Singh and S. S. Jamil. Phytochemical and Pharmacological profile of Withania somnifera Dunal: a review. Journal of Applied and Pharmaceutical Science (2012) 2(1): 170-175.

15   Animesh K. Datta, Ananya Das, Arnab Bhattacharya, Suchetana Mukherjee, Benoy K, Ghosh. An overview on Withania somnifera (L) Dunal- The Indian ginseng. Medicinal and Aromatic Plant Science and Biotechnology (2011) 5 (1): 1-15.

16   S. K. Kulakarni, Ashish Dhir. Withania somnifera: An Indian ginseng.

Progress in Neuro-Psychopharmacology & Biological Psychiatry (2008) 32: 1093-1105.

17 Vikas Kumar, Amitabha Dey, Mallinath B. Hadimani, Tatjana Marcovic, Mila Emerald. Chemistry and Pharmacology of Withania somnifera: An update. TANG (2015) 5 (1): 1-12.

18 Mohammad Hossein Mirjalili, Elisabeth Moyano, Mercedes Bonfill, Rosa M. Cusido and Javier Palazon. Steroidal lactones from Withania somnifera, an ancient plant for novel medicine. Molecules (2009) 14: 2373-2393.

19 Khaula Shirin, Saima Imad, Sheraz Shafiq, Kaneez Fatima. Determination of major and trace elements in the indigenous medicinal plant Withania somnifera and their possible correlation with therapeutic activity. Journal of Saudi Chemical Society (2010) 14: 97-100.

20 Harish Chandra Andola, Vijay Kant Purohit. High performance thin layer chromatography (HPTLC): a modern analytical tool for biological analysis. Nature and Science (2010) 8 (10): 58-61.

21 Vivek Sharma, Ajai P. Gupta, Pamita Bhandari, Raghbir C. Gupta, Bikram Singh. A validated and densitometric HPTLC method for the quantification of Withaferin A and Withanolide A in different plant parts of two morphotypes of Withania somnifera. Chromatographia (2007) 66 (9/10): 801-804.

22 Neha Narendrabhai Mistry, Purvi Shah, Kalpana Patel, Lal Hingorani. Simultaneous estimation of stigmasterol and Withaferin A in union total herbal formulation using validated HPTLC method. Journal of Applied Pharmaceutical Science (2015) 5 (8): 159-166.

23 Jay Savai, Nancy Pandita and Meena Chintamaneni. Simultaneous determination & validation of two different withanolides in Withania somnifera using various chromatographic techniques. Indo American Journal of Pharmaceutical Research (2014) 4 (11): 5449-5458.

24 Supriya S. Jirge, Pratima A. Tatke and Satish Y. Gabhe. Development and validation of a novel HPTLC method for simultaneous estimation of beta-sitosterol-D-glucoside and Withaferin A. International Journal of Pharmacy and Pharmaceutical Sciences (2011) 3 (2): 227-230.

25 Safeena Sheikh, Suhail Asghar, Showkat Ahmad. Development and validation of method for the estimation of Withanolide A from herbal oral thin film. International Journal of Innovative Research & Development (2013) 2 (1): 171-180.

26 Deepak Mundkinajeddu, Laxman P. Sawant, Rojison Koshy, Praneetha Akunuri, Vineet Kumar Singh, Anand Mayachari, Maged H. M. Sharaf, Murali Balasubramanian, and Amit Agarwal. Development and validation of high performance liquid chromatography method for simultaneous estimation of flavonoid glycosides in Withania somnifera aerial parts. ISRN Analytical Chemistry, Volume 2014, Article ID 351547, 6 pages.

27 Shaila Dalavayi, S. M. Kulkarni, Rajya Lakshmi Itikala, S. Itikala. Determination of Withaferin A in two Withania species by RP-HPLC. Indian Journal of Pharmaceutical Sciences (2006) 68 (2): 253-256.

28 Rathod B and Kilambi P. Development of validated RP-HPLC method for the estimation of Withaferin A in Withania somnifera, its extract and polyherbal formulations. Pharma Science Monitor (2013) 4 (3): 1-9.

29 Hafsa Ahmad, Kiran Khandelwal, Shakti Deep Pachauri, Rajender Singh Sanghwan, Anil Kumar Dwivedi. Stability indicating studies on NMITLI 118 RT+ (standardized extract of Withania somnifera Dunal). Pharmacognosy Magazine (2014) 10 (39): 227-233.

30 J. V. Manwar, K. R. Mahadik, A. R. Paradkar, S. P. Takle, L. Sathiyanarayanan and S. V. Patil. Determination of withanolides from the

roots and herbal formulation of Withania somnifera by HPLC using DAD and ELSD detector. Der Pharmacia sinica (2012) 3 (1); 41-46.

31 M. Ganzera, M. I. Choudhary, I. A. Khan. Quantitative HPLC analysis of withanolides in Withania somnifera. Fitoterapia (2003) 74: 68-76.

32 Vivek Sharma. HPLC – PDA method for quantification of Withaferin A and Withanolide A in diploid (n=12) and tetraploid (n=24) cytotypes of " Indian Ginseng" Withania somnifera (L.) Dunal from north India. International Journal of Indigenous Medicinal Plants (2013) 46 (2): 1245-1250.

33 N. Gurav, B. Solanki, I. Gadhvi, P. Patel and D. Sen. RP-HPLC method development and validation for estimation of Withaferin A in Ranger capsule. International Journal of Pharmaceutical Sciences and Research (2015) 6 (12): 5141-5146.

2 – Antioxidant Activity

2.1 – Antioxidant

An antioxidant is "any substance that when present at low concentration relative to an oxidizable substrate, prevents or significantly delays oxidation of the substrate"[1]. Antioxidants are well known for their ability to defend the body against free radical damage.

2.2 – Free Radicals

A free radical is a chemical entity that contains one or more unpaired electrons. Free radicals are highly reactive. The term reactive oxygen species (ROS) refers to oxygen-containing radicals as well as some non-radical derivatives that contain oxygen. Examples of ROS include hydroxyl ($HO^{\bullet}$), superoxide ($O_2^{\bullet-}$), peroxyl ($RO_2^{\bullet}$) and singlet oxygen (Δg). An analogous term, reactive nitrogen species (RNS), is used for nitrogen-containing radicals and non-radical derivatives. Examples of RNS include nitric oxide ($NO^{\bullet}$), nitrogen dioxide ($NO_2^{\bullet}$), nitrous acid (HNO_2) and peroxynitrite ($ONOO^-$).

2.3 – Formation and sources of Free Radicals

Free radicals are generally formed by homolytic bond dissociation or single-electron oxidation of an atom or molecule:

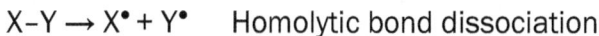

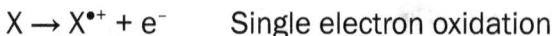

$$X–Y \rightarrow X^{\bullet} + Y^{\bullet} \quad \text{Homolytic bond dissociation}$$

$$X \rightarrow X^{\bullet+} + e^- \quad \text{Single electron oxidation}$$

Free radicals are present almost everywhere. We are exposed to free radicals from both exogenous and endogenous sources. Exogenous sources include radiation, pollution, cigarette smoke, alcohol, processed food, xenobiotics, pathogens and others[2]. Free radicals are constantly produced in the body as byproducts of biochemical processes at various cellular locations. Mitochondria are considered to be the largest source of ROS[3]. Mitochondria consume 80-90% of cellular oxygen to support oxidative phosphorylation, the metabolic pathway that harnesses energy released by the oxidation of nutrients to produce adenosine triphosphate (ATP). In this process, oxygen (O_2) undergoes a four-electron reduction to water:

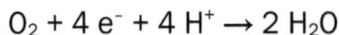

$$O_2 + 4\ e^- + 4\ H^+ \rightarrow 2\ H_2O$$

During this process, partial reduction of oxygen also occurs, producing superoxide ($O_2^{\bullet-}$)[4]. It is estimated that 0.1-2% of the oxygen consumed by mitochondria is partially reduced to superoxide[3,4,5]. Superoxide is converted to hydrogen peroxide (H_2O_2) by spontaneous dismutation or by superoxide dismutase (SOD). In the presence of metal ions, H_2O_2 is converted to the hydroxyl radical ($HO^\bullet$)[6]. In addition to mitochondria, there are other endogenous sources of ROS/RNS[2].

2.4 – Free Radical Reactions

Free radicals are highly reactive. Lipid membranes, proteins, carbohydrates and DNA are highly susceptible to free radical attack[7-11]. Lipid membranes contain phospholipids, essential components of which are polyunsaturated fatty acids (PUFAs). PUFAs are highly susceptible to oxidation due to their double bonds. This type of oxidation, lipid peroxidation (LPO), is a chain reaction consisting of three steps: chain initiation, chain propagation and chain termination. LPO produces a variety of toxic products such as 4-hydroxy-2-nonenal (4-HNE), malondialdehyde (MDA), 2-propenal (acrolein) and isoprostane. LPO impairs membrane functions, reduces fluidity, inactivates membrane receptors and enzymes, and increases non-specific permeability of ions[12]. Free radical attack on proteins can cause peroxidation, fragmentation, damage to amino acids and alteration to tertiary structure[7,13]. Free radical attack on DNA can cause strand breaks, DNA-DNA and DNA-protein cross-linking, DNA base and sugar modification, and loss of purines[7]. Free radicals have been implicated in several diseases and the aging process[2,14].

2.5 – Oxidative Stress and the Antioxidant Defense System

Oxidative stress has been defined as an imbalance between oxidants and antioxidants in favor of the former[15]. While too much oxidative stress is harmful, too little oxidative stress is also unfavorable. Free radicals are beneficial at certain levels. To ward off free radical damage, humans and other aerobic organisms have developed integrated antioxidant defense systems. The first line of defense includes preventive antioxidants that suppress the formation of free radicals. The second line of defense includes radical scavenging antioxidants that remove free radicals before they can cause damage. The third line of defense consists of enzymes that can repair damage to proteins, DNA, oxidized lipids, etc. The body's adaptation mechanism acts as the fourth line of defense. Both endogenous and exogenous components help maintain the body's antioxidant defense system[16].

2.6 – In Vitro Evidence for Antioxidant Activity

2.6.1 – Diphenyl picrylhydrazyl (DPPH) Scavenging Activity

This method, originally proposed by Blois[17], is widely used to assay the antioxidant activity of plant drugs. An alcoholic solution of DPPH has a purple color and absorbs light strongly at around 520 nm. Adding an antioxidant changes the color to yellow and decreases the absorbance at 520 nm. The decrease in absorbance is considered to be proportional to the free radical scavenging activity of the added antioxidant. The results from several studies using this method to evaluate the antioxidant activity of Withania somnifera are summarized below (Table 2.1).

Extract and standard	Results	Ref
Extract: methanol **Standard:** trolox	methanol extract and trolox scavenged DPPH in a dose-dependent manner (50-400 µg/ml)	18
Extracts: aqueous extracts of leaves, fresh tubers and dry tubers	leaves > fresh tubers > dry tubers	19
Extract: methanol extract of root **Standard:** ascorbic acid	IC_{50} (mg/ml): methanol=11.28, ascorbic acid=3.46	20
Extract: aqueous extract of root	IC_{50} = 524 µg/ml	21
Extracts: Methanol-water (4:1) extracts of different parts	stellar part of mature root > young root bark > bark of mature root > senescent leaf > fruits > mature leaf > young stem > immature leaf > stellar part of young root > calyx	22
Extracts: methanol (80%) extracts of root (WSREt), fruit (WSFEt) and leaves (WSLEt)	WSLEt > WSFEt > WSREt	23

Extracts: root was sequentially extracted with hexane, chloroform, ethyl acetate, acetone, methanol and water **Standard:** BHA	IC_{50} (µg/ml): BHA=13, methanol=56, water=94, ethyl acetate=115, acetone=194, chloroform=283, hexane=404	24
Extracts: ethanol and water extracts of root **Standard:** ascorbic acid	IC_{50} (µg/ml): ethanol=14.5, ascorbic acid=15.6	25
Extracts: methanol (80%) extracts of roots (WSREt), leaves (WSLEt) and fruits (WSFEt) **Standards:** ascorbic acid, BHT	IC_{50} (µg/ml): ascorbic acid=26, BHT=38, WSLEt=101.7, WSFEt=345.7, WSREt=801.9	26
Extract: methanol-water (7:3) extract of root **Standard:** ascorbic acid	IC_{50} (µg/ml): ascorbic acid=5.3, extract=650.4	27
Extracts: root powder was successively extracted with petroleum ether, n-hexane, ethanol, chloroform and methanol **Standards:** ascorbic acid, BHT	IC_{50} (µg/ml): ascorbic acid=5.7, BHT=8.8, chloroform=87, petroleum ether=145, methanol=268, ethanol=529	28
Extracts: ethanol, ethanol-water (1:9) and water extracts of roots obtained by using soxhlet (SOX), ultrasound-assisted solvent extraction (UASE) and microwave-assisted solvent extraction (MASE)	ethanol > ethanol-water > water UASE and MASE were found to be viable alternatives to traditional extraction	29
Extracts: methanol (80%) and water extracts of root **Standard:** BHT	IC_{50} (mg/ml): BHT=0.56, methanol=2.9, water=3.27	30
Extracts: petroleum ether, chloroform and methanol extracts of root	methanol > chloroform > petroleum ether	31
Extract: ethanol-water (70:30) extract of root **Standard:** ascorbic acid	IC_{50} (µg/ml): ascorbic acid=15, extract=352	32
Extracts: ethanol-water (50:50), methanol and water extracts of root **Standard:** ascorbic acid	ascorbic acid > ethanol-water > methanol > water	33

Extract: root powder was extracted successively with petroleum ether and methanol. methanol extract was used. Standard: ascorbic acid	IC$_{50}$ (μg/ml): ascorbic acid=57.6, methanol=65.84	34
Extract: methanol extract of root Standard: ascorbic acid	IC$_{50}$ (μg/ml): ascorbic acid=8, methanol=27.8	35
Extracts: methanol (99.5%), acetone, ethyl acetate (99.7%) and chloroform extracts of leaf, stem and root Standard: ascorbic acid	ascorbic acid > chloroform > methanol > acetone > ethyl acetate root extracts showed greater activity than others	36
Extract: ethanol extract of root (EEWS) Standards: α-tocopherol, ascorbic acid, BHA, BHT	EEWS > BHA > ascorbic acid > BHT > α-tocopherol	37
Extracts: water and ethanol extracts of leaf	IC$_{50}$ (μg/ml): water=1445, ethanol=1663	38
Extracts: leaf powder was sequentially extracted with hexane, chloroform, ethyl acetate, acetone, methanol and water Standard: BHA	IC$_{50}$ (μg/ml): BHA=10, methanol=200, water=240, ethyl acetate=280, acetone=400, chloroform=480, hexane=720	39
Extract: root powder was defatted with petroleum ether and extracted with methanol Standard: ascorbic acid	IC$_{50}$ (μg/ml): ascorbic acid=10, extract=12	40

Table 2.1: DPPH radical scavenging activity of Withania somnifera

2.6.2 – Superoxide ($O_2^{\bullet-}$) Scavenging Activity

The most important physiological source of superoxide is mitochondria[3,41-43]. There are various other sources as well. Superoxide gets converted to H_2O_2 by spontaneous dismutation or by the enzyme superoxide dismutase. In the presence of metal ions, highly reactive hydroxyl radicals are produced by the Fenton or Haber-Weiss reactions[6]. Superoxide reacts with nitric oxide to produce the highly reactive peroxynitrite. Various extracts of Withania somnifera have been shown to scavenge superoxide and the results are summarized below (Table 2.2).

Extract and Standard	Results	Ref
Extract: methanol	showed dose-dependent superoxide scavenging activity (3-25 µg/ml)	18
Extracts: root powder was successively extracted with hexane, chloroform, ethyl acetate, acetone, methanol and water **Standard:** BHA	IC_{50} (µg/ml): BHA=40, methanol=94, water=125, ethyl acetate=148, acetone=168, chloroform=178, hexane=740	24
Extracts: Ethanol extract of root (EEWS) **Standard:** α-tocopherol, Ascorbic acid, BHA and BHT	BHT > α-tocopherol > ascorbic acid > BHA > EEWS	37
Extracts: Leaf powder was sequentially extracted with hexane, chloroform, ethyl acetate, acetone, methanol and water **Standard:** BHA	IC_{50} (ug/ml): BHA=25, methanol=80, ethyl acetate=130, water=150, acetone=200, chloroform=225, hexane=550	39
Extract: water	showed dose-dependent superoxide scavenging activity (100-200 µg/ml)	44
Extracts: methanol-water (80:20) and water extracts	IC_{50} (mg/ml): methanol-water=34.3, water=36.6	30
Extract: root powder was defatted with petroleum ether and extracted with methanol **Standard:** ascorbic acid	IC_{50} extract=19 ug/ml (close to standard)	40
Extract: ethanol and water extracts of leaf	IC_{50} (µg/ml): water=1352, ethanol=1597	38

Table 2.2: Superoxide scavenging activity of Withania somnifera

2.6.3 – Anti-lipid Peroxidation Activity

Lipid peroxidation is very likely to occur if reactive free radicals are formed in biological tissues where PUFAs are abundant. Free radical-mediated lipid peroxidation is implicated in the pathogenesis of a number of diseases[45,46]. The most common method for screening and monitoring LPO is the thiobarbituric acid reactive substances (TBARS) assay. This method is based on the reaction of two molecules of thiobarbituric acid (TBA) and one molecule of malondialdehyde (MDA), a byproduct of LPO, to produce an adduct that absorbs at 532 nm[45]. The use of antioxidants to inhibit LPO has received considerable attention. A number of in vitro studies have evaluated the anti-LPO activity of Withania somnifera and the results are summarized below (Table 2.3).

Extract and Standard	Results	Ref
Extracts: water extracts of leaves, fresh tubers and dry tubers	All extracts inhibited H_2O_2-induced LPO in goat liver homogenate leaves > fresh tubers > dry tubers	19
Extract: methanol extract of root **Standard:** ascorbic acid	extract inhibited $FeCl_3$-induced LPO in rat liver homogenate; extract effect was slightly smaller than ascorbic acid	20
Extract: water extract of root	extract inhibited $FeSO_4$-induced LPO in rat liver homogenate (IC_{50} = 270 µg/ml)	21
Extracts: methanol-water (4:1) extracts of various parts	all extracts inhibited $FeSO_4$-induced LPO in goat liver homogenate bark of mature root > senescent leaf > fruits > mature leaf > young root bark > stellar part of mature root > calyx > young stem > immature leaf > stellar part of young root	22
Extract: methanol water (7:3) extract of root **Standard:** trolox	extract inhibited LPO in brain homogenate of mice induced by $FeSO_4$/ascorbic acid. IC_{50} (µg/ml): trolox=13.5, extract=284	27
Extracts: root powder was sequentially extracted with hexane, chloroform, ethyl acetate, acetone, methanol and water **Standard:** BHA	all extracts inhibited $FeSO_4$-induced LPO in egg yolk homogenate. IC_{50} (mg/ml): BHA=0.2, water=0.5, methanol=0.5, ethyl acetate=0.72, acetone=0.93, chloroform=1.2, hexane=3.04	47
Extracts: ethanol-water (50:50), methanol and water extracts of root	all extracts inhibited $FeCl_3$-induced LPO in rat liver homogenate ethanol-water > methanol > water	33
Extract: ethanol (70%) extract of root	extract inhibited $FeSO_4$-induced LPO in rat heart homogenate in a dose-dependent manner (100-500 µg/ml) IC_{50} = 226 µg/ml	48
Extracts: leaf was sequentially extracted with hexane, chloroform, ethyl acetate, acetone, methanol and water **Standard:** BHA	all extracts inhibited $FeSO_4$-induced LPO in egg yolk homogenate. IC_{50} (µg/ml): BHA=20, methanol=540, water=650, ethyl acetate=750, acetone=940, chloroform=1120, hexane=2480	39

Table 2.3: Anti-Lipid peroxidation activity of Withania somnifera

2.6.4 – Fe^{2+} Chelating Activity

In the presence of Fe^{2+}, H_2O_2 is converted into the highly reactive hydroxyl radical. Removal of Fe^{2+} by chelation makes it unavailable for hydroxyl generation. A number of studies have demonstrated the Fe^{2+} chelating activity of Withania somnifera and the results are summarized below (Table 2.4).

Extract and standard	Results	Ref
Extracts: methanol (80%) extracts of root (WSREt), leaf (WSLEt) and fruit (WSFEt) **Standard:** EDTA	IC_{50} (mg/ml): EDTA=0.1, WSLEt=0.2, WSREt=0.4, WSFEt=0.7	26
Extracts: root powder was sequentially extracted with hexane, chloroform, ethyl acetate, acetone, methanol and water **Standard:** EDTA	IC_{50} (µg/ml): EDTA=10, methanol=70, water=94, ethyl acetate=114, acetone=145, chloroform=163, hexane=626	24
Extracts: methanol (99.5%), acetone, ethyl acetate (99.7%) and chloroform extracts of leaf, stem and root **Standard:** ascorbic acid	all extracts showed Fe^{2+} chelating ability; root extracts showed the highest chelating activity and were similar to the standard	36
Extracts: leaf powder was sequentially extracted with hexane, chloroform, ethyl acetate, acetone, methanol and water **Standard:** EDTA	IC_{50} (µg/ml): EDTA=<10, methanol=65, ethyl acetate=80, acetone=90, water=120, chloroform=200, hexane=590	39
Extract: root powder was defatted with petroleum ether and extracted with methanol **Standard:** ascorbic acid	IC_{50} (µg/ml): ascorbic acid=17, extract=18	40
Extract: ethanol extract of root (EEWS) **Standards:** α-tocopherol, ascorbic acid, BHA, BHT	EEWS > BHA > ascorbic acid > BHT > α-tocopherol	37

Table 2.4: Fe^{2+} chelating activity of Withania somnifera

2.6.5 – Nitric Oxide Scavenging Activity

Nitric oxide is generated by the oxidation of arginine catalyzed by various nitric oxide synthase enzymes[7]. During the oxidative burst triggered by the inflammation process, the immune system produces both superoxide and nitric oxide. Nitric oxide mediates a number of diverse physiological processes including vasodilation, smooth muscle relaxation, neurotransmission and immune system regulation. Improper control of nitric oxide levels causes diverse pathologies[49]. A number of investigations have shown the nitric oxide scavenging activity of Withania somnifera and the results are summarized below (Table 2.5).

Extract and standard	Results	Ref
Extract: water extract of root	showed dose-dependent nitric oxide scavenging activity (IC_{50} = 7.6 µg/ml)	21
Extract: methanol-water extract (7:3) of root **Standard:** curcumin	IC_{50} (µg/ml): curcumin=91, extract=406	27
Extracts: root powder was sequentially extracted with hexane, chloroform, ethyl acetate, acetone, methanol and water **Standard:** ascorbic acid	IC_{50} (mg/ml): ascorbic acid=1.8, methanol=3.8, acetone=4.8, ethyl acetate=5.1, water=5.5, chloroform=7.4, hexane=10.4	47
Extract: root powder was successively extracted with petroleum ether, n-hexane, ethanol, chloroform and methanol **Standards:** BHT, ascorbic acid	IC_{50} (µg/ml): BHT=27, ascorbic acid=28, chloroform=92, petroleum ether=289, methanol=449, ethanol=719, n-hexane=847	28
Extract: ethanol-water (70:30) extract of root **Standard:** ascorbic acid	scavenged nitric oxide in a dose-dependent manner (2-1000 µg/ml) IC_{50} (µg/ml): ascorbic acid=17, extract=378	32
Extract: root powder was defatted with petroleum ether and extracted with methanol	IC_{50} = 27 µg/ml	40

Table 2.5: Nitric oxide scavenging activity of Withania somnifera

2.6.6 – Hydroxyl Radical Scavenging Activity

Hydroxyl radicals are generated in the body by the Fenton reaction[6]. Hydroxyl radicals are highly reactive and can attack most organic and inorganic molecules in cells including DNA, proteins, lipids, amino acids and sugars[2,7]. A number of in vitro studies have shown the hydroxyl radical scavenging activity of Withania somnifera and the results are summarized below (Table 2.6).

Extract and Standard	Results	Ref
Extract: methanol extract of root **Standard:** ascorbic acid	extract showed slightly lower scavenging activity than the standard	20
Extracts: root was successively extracted with hexane, chloroform, ethyl acetate, acetone, methanol and water **Standard:** gallic acid	IC_{50} (mg/ml): gallic acid=0.30, methanol=0.57, water=0.80, acetone=1.23, ethyl acetate=1.36, chloroform=2.12, hexane=9.33	24
Extract: methanol-water (7:3) extract of root. **Standard:** Mannitol	IC_{50} (µg/ml): standard=580, extract=1808	27
Extracts: leaf powder was extracted sequentially with hexane, chloroform, ethyl acetate, acetone, methanol and water **Standard:** gallic acid	all extracts scavenged hydroxyl radicals; methanol showed the highest activity ($IC_{50} \approx 790$ µg/ml) and hexane showed the lowest activity ($IC_{50} \approx 7000$ µg/ml) IC_{50} of gallic acid was less than 200 µg/ml	39

Table 2.6: Hydroxyl radical scavenging activity of Withania somnifera

2.6.7 – Hydrogen Peroxide Scavenging Activity

Hydrogen peroxide is produced by the dismutation of superoxide catalyzed by superoxide dismutase[7]. Hydrogen peroxide is a non-radical ROS and can cause damage directly and indirectly. Its direct damage includes degradation of heme proteins, inactivation of enzymes and oxidation of DNA, lipids, -SH groups and keto acids. Indirect damage includes conversion of hydrogen peroxide to other highly reactive radicals. A number of investigations have shown the hydrogen peroxide scavenging activity of Withania somnifera and some results are presented below (Table 2.7).

Extract and Standard	Results	Ref
Extracts: root powder was successively extracted with hexane, chloroform, ethyl acetate, acetone, methanol and water **Standard:** ascorbic acid	IC_{50} (mg/ml): ascorbic acid=0.16, methanol=0.29, water=0.32, acetone=2.13, ethyl acetate=2.5, chloroform=3.85, hexane=6.62	24
Extracts: root powder was successively extracted with petroleum ether, n-hexane, ethanol, chloroform and methanol **Standards:** BHT, ascorbic acid	IC_{50} (µg/ml): BHT=6.39, ascorbic acid=7.53, chloroform=89.19, petroleum ether=162.64, methanol=172.66, ethanol=327.51, n-hexane=753.19	28
Extract: root powder was defatted with petroleum ether and extracted with methanol. **Standard:** ascorbic acid	IC_{50} (µg/ml): standard=36, extract=64	40
Extract: ethanol extract of root (EEWS) **Standards:** BHA, ascorbic acid, BHT, α-tocopherol	EEWS > BHA > ascorbic acid > BHT > α-tocopherol	37

Table 2.7: Hydrogen peroxide scavenging activity of Withania somnifera

2.6.8 – ABTS$^{•+}$ [2-2'-azino-bis-(3-ethyl-benzothiazoline-6-sulphonic acid] Radical Scavenging Activity

This assay is based on the interaction between the antioxidant and the ABTS$^{•+}$ radical cation. ABTS$^{•+}$ is generated by reacting ABTS with a strong oxidizing agent like potassium persulfate. ABTS$^{•+}$ absorbs light at 734 nm[50]. Reduction of ABTS$^{•+}$ by an antioxidant decreases the absorbance; this can be used to estimate the antioxidant capacity. A number of studies have used this method to estimate the antioxidant capacity of Withania somnifera and some results are presented below (Table 2.8).

Extract and Standard	Results	Ref
Extracts: ethanol, ethanol–water (1:9) and water extracts; prepared by soxhlet (SOX) extraction, Ultrasound-assisted solvent extraction (UASE), and microwave-assisted solvent extraction (MASE)	water > ethanol-water > ethanol	29
Extract: aqueous methanol and water extracts **Standard:** trolox	IC_{50} (mg/ml): aqueous methanol=28.35, water=32.55, trolox=428.38	30
Extract: root powder was successively extracted with petroleum ether and methanol; methanol extract was used **Standard:** ascorbic acid	IC_{50} (µg/ml): extract=4.63, standard=5.35	34
Extract: root powder was defatted with petroleum ether and extracted with methanol **Standard:** ascorbic acid	IC_{50} (µg/ml): standard=16, extract=18	40

Table 2.8: ABTS$^{\bullet+}$ Radical scavenging activity of Withania somnifera

2.7 – In Vivo Studies

A number of in vivo studies have been conducted to determine the antioxidant activity of Withania somnifera and the results from some publications are summarized below.

Panda and Kar[51] found that treating Swiss albino mice with Withania somnifera root powder (0.7 or 1.4 g/kg/day, gastric intubation) for 30 days decreased LPO and increased SOD and CAT in the liver compared to controls.

Bhattacharya and coworkers[52] showed that treating adult male Wistar rats with glycowithanolides extracted from Withania somnifera (WSG, 10 or 20 mg/kg/day, i.p.) for 14 or 21 days increased the activities of SOD, CAT and GPx in the frontal cortex and striatum compared to controls. The effect of WSG (20 mg) was comparable to the standard drug (-) deprenyl (2 mg/kg/day, i.p.). Another investigation[53] evaluated the effect of WSG on stress-induced oxidative stress in the rat brain. Adult male Wistar rats were treated with the vehicle or WSG (10-50 mg/kg/day, P.O.) for 21 days. Each day, the animals were given foot shocks one hour after the treatment. The control group received the vehicle and was not subjected to stress. Rats treated with the vehicle and subjected to stress showed increased LPO and SOD accompanied by decreased GPx and CAT in the frontal cortex and striatum compared to the control group. Rats treated with WSG and subjected to stress showed a reversal of these changes. The authors concluded that "The results of the present study indicate that the anti-stress adaptogenic activity of WSG may be, at least in part, due to its antioxidant effect".

Dhule[54] investigated the effect of an aqueous extract of Withania somnifera roots (WS) on lipid peroxidation (LPO) in stressed animals. Male rabbits and mice were treated with lipopolysaccharide (LPS, 0.2 mg/kg, intravenous) from Klebsiella pneumoniae or peptidoglycan (PGN 100 mg/kg, intravenous) from Staphylococcus aureus. Both rabbits and mice showed increased blood LPO. Oral administration of WS (100 mg/kg) prevented the elevation of LPO.

Parihar and Hemnani[55] showed that an extract of Withania somnifera mitigated the oxidative changes induced by kainic acid (KA) in the mouse hippocampus. An acetone extract of Withania somnifera roots was fractionated with methanol:hexane (1:1). The dried methanol fraction (WSMF) was reconstituted in aqueous ethanol (12% v/v) and used in the study. Female Swiss albino mice treated with KA (0.25 μg in 0.5 ml, intrahippocampal injection) showed increased LPO and PC and decreased GPx and GSH in the hippocampus compared to controls. Mice treated with WSMF (20 mg/kg/day, P.O.) for 3 weeks and injected with KA showed a reversal of these changes.

Khanam and Devi[56] reported that Swiss albino mice treated with lead nitrate (40 mg/kg, i.p.) showed decreased SOD, CAT and GSH in the liver compared to controls. Mice treated with a methanol extract of Withania somnifera roots (250 mg/kg/day, P.O.) for 7 days followed by lead nitrate showed increased SOD, CAT and GSH in the liver compared to the lead nitrate-only group.

Anwer and coworkers[57] found that diabetic Swiss albino Wistar rats showed increased LPO and decreased activities of GPx, GR, GST, SOD and CAT in pancreatic tissue compared to controls. Treatment of NIDDM rats with an aqueous extract of Withania somnifera roots reversed the oxidative changes.

Naidu and coworkers[58] reported that male Wistar rats treated with reserpine (1 mg/kg/day, SC) on alternate days for three days (days 1, 3 and 5) showed increased LPO and decreased GSH, CAT and SOD in the brain compared to controls. Rats treated with reserpine for three alternate days followed by treatment with a Withania somnifera root extract (50 or 100 mg/kg/day, P.O.) for 4 weeks reversed these changes.

Visavadiya and Narasimhacharya[59] examined the antioxidant effect of Withania somnifera root powder (WS) in hypercholesteremic rats. Hypercholesteremia was induced by feeding rats a special diet containing 0.5 g % cholesterol and 1.0 g % sodium taurocholate. Charles Foster male rats (3 months old) treated with the special diet for 4 weeks showed increased hepatic LPO and decreased SOD, CAT and ascorbic acid compared to controls. Rats treated with a special diet containing WS (0.75 g % or 1.5 g %) for 4 weeks reversed the oxidative changes.

Rajasankar and coworkers[60] showed that an extract of Withania somnifera (WS) reversed the oxidative changes induced by MPTP (1-methyl-4-phenyl-1,2,3,6–tetrahydropyridine) in the mouse brain. Male Swiss albino mice treated with MPTP (20 mg/kg/day, i.p.) for 4 days showed increased MDA, SOD and CAT and decreased GPx and GSH in the midbrain and striatum compared to controls. Mice treated with WS (100 mg/kg/day, P.O.) for 3 days followed by treatment with MPTP and WS for 4 days showed a reversal of these changes.

Kumar and Kumar[61] investigated the effect of Withania somnifera root extract (WS) on 3-nitropropionic acid (3-NP)-induced oxidative stress in the rat brain. Male Wistar rats treated with 3-NP (10 mg/kg/day, i.p.) for 14 days showed increased LPO and nitrite and decreased SOD and CAT in the striatum and cortex compared to controls. Rats treated with WS (100 mg/kg/day, P.O.) followed by 3-NP treatment for 14 days showed a reversal of these changes.

Udayakumar and coworkers[62] demonstrated the antioxidant effect of ethanol (80%) extracts of Withania somnifera roots (WSREt) and leaves (WSLEt) in diabetic rats. Male adult albino Wistar rats were injected with alloxan monohydrate (150 mg/kg, i.p.) dissolved in saline to induce diabetes. Normal healthy rats were used as controls. Diabetic rats showed increased LPO and decreased SOD, CAT, GPx, GSH and GST in the liver and decreased vitamin C and E in plasma compared to controls. Diabetic rats treated with WSREt, WSLEt or glibenclamide showed decreased LPO and increased SOD, CAT, GPx, GSH and GST in the liver and increased vitamin C and E compared to untreated diabetic rats.

Sharma and coworkers[63] reported the antioxidant effect of a methanol-water (80:20) extract of Withania somnifera roots (WS) against lead nitrate-induced oxidative stress in the mouse brain. Male Swiss albino mice treated with lead nitrate (20 mg/kg/day, via oral gavage) for 42 days showed increased LPO and decreased

SOD, CAT, GSH and GST in the brain compared to controls. Mice treated with lead nitrate+WS (200 or 400 mg/kg/day, via oral gavage) showed a reversal of these changes to near control levels.

Soman and coworkers[64] investigated the antioxidant effect of an aqueous extract of Withania somnifera roots (WSR) and withanolide A (WLA) in epileptic rats. Epilepsy was induced in male Wistar rats by injecting pilocarpine. Epileptic rats showed increased LPO and decreased SOD and CAT in the hippocampus compared to non-epileptic controls. Epileptic rats treated with WSR (100 mg/kg/day, P.O.) or WLA (10 μmol/kg/day, P.O.) for 15 days showed decreased LPO and increased SOD and CAT compared to untreated epileptic rats.

Patil and coworkers[65] reported the antioxidant activity of an alcohol extract of Withania somnifera leaves (WSLF) in galactose-stressed mice. Male mice treated with D-galactose showed increased LPO in the testis and epididymis compared to controls. Mice treated with D-galactose+WSLF showed decreased LPO in the testis and epididymis compared to D-galactose-only mice.

Baitharu and coworkers[66] demonstrated that an extract of Withania somnifera roots (WSRT) attenuated oxidative stress in the rat hippocampus induced by hypobaric hypoxia (HH). The extract contained significant amounts of Withaferin A, Withanolide A and Withanolide D. Adult male Sprague Dawley rats exposed to HH for 7 days showed increased ROS and LPO and decreased GSH and SOD in the hippocampus compared to controls. Rats treated with WSRT (200 mg/kg/day, via feeding cannula) for 21 days followed by exposure to HH along with WSRT treatment for the next 7 days showed decreased ROS and LPO and increased GSH and SOD in the hippocampus compared to untreated rats exposed to HH.

Manjunath and Muralidhara[67] reported that an extract of Withania somnifera roots (Withanolides, 2.57%; Withaferin A, 2.38%) mitigated oxidative stress induced by rotenone (RT) in Drosophila melanogaster. Whole-body homogenate of Drosophila melanogaster flies exposed to RT and simultaneously treated with the extract showed decreased LPO, ROS and HP and increased GSH, SOD, CAT, and GST compared to the homogenate from untreated flies exposed to RT.

Ahmed and coworkers[68] examined the effect of a standardized extract of Withania somnifera (withaferin 0.232% w/w) on oxidative stress induced by intracerebroventricular injections of streptozotocin (ICV-STZ) in rats. Male Wistar rats treated with the extract (100-300 mg/kg/day, P.O.) for 3 weeks and infused bilaterally with ICV-STZ injections (3 mg/kg) in normal saline showed decreased LPO and increased GSH, GPX, GR and CAT compared to ICV-STZ-injected rats not treated with the extract.

Jasuja and coworkers[69] reported that a methanol (70%) extract of Withania somnifera leaves and roots attenuated oxidative changes induced by acephate (an organophosphate) in rats. Male albino rats treated with acephate (75 mg/kg/day, P.O.) for 15 days showed increased LPO and decreased GSH, CAT and SOD in the testis compared to controls. Rats treated with acephate for 15 days followed by the extract (100 mg/kg/day, P.O.) for the next 15 days showed decreased LPO and increased GSH, CAT and SOD in the testis compared to acephate-only rats.

Malik and coworkers[70] evaluated the antioxidant activity of an aqueous extract of Withania somnifera roots (WS) on paracetamol (PCM)-induced oxidative stress in the mouse liver. Female Swiss albino mice treated with PCM (500 mg/kg/day via oral gavage) for 28 days showed increased LPO and decreased CAT, GR, GPx and GSH in the liver compared to controls. Mice treated with PCM along with WS (500 mg/kg/day, P.O.) for 28 days showed decreased LPO and increased CAT, GR, GPx and GSH compared to PCM-only mice.

Chopra and coworkers[71] evaluated the antioxidant effect of an aqueous extract of Withania somnifera on oxidative stress induced by cadmium in the mouse spleen. BALB/c mice injected with cadmium sulfate (5 mg/kg/day, i.p.) for 5 days showed increased LPO and decreased GSH, GST, CAT and SOD in the spleen compared to controls. Mice treated with cadmium sulfate+extract (500 mg/kg/day, P.O.) for 5 days showed decreased LPO and increased GSH, GST, CAT and SOD in the spleen compared to cadmium sulfate-only mice.

Sabina and coworkers[72] reported the antioxidant activity of Withania somnifera against paracetamol (PCM)-induced oxidative stress in rats. Rats treated with PCM (900 mg/kg, i.p.) showed decreased serum SOD, CAT, GST and GSH compared to controls. Rats treated with PCM followed by an aqueous suspension of Withania somnifera (500 or 1000 mg/kg, P.O.) showed increased serum SOD, CAT, GST and GSH compared to PCM-only rats. The effect of Withania somnifera was comparable to silymarin (25 mg/kg, i.p.)

Vedi and coworkers[73] demonstrated the antioxidant effect of Withania somnifera root powder against bromobenzene-induced oxidative stress in rats. Wistar albino rats treated with bromobenzene (10 mmol/kg in 0.1 ml coconut oil, via intragastric tube) showed increased LPO and decreased CAT, SOD, GST, GPx and GSH in plasma and liver tissues compared to controls. Rats treated with

Withania somnifera for 8 days followed by treatment with bromobenzene on day 8 showed a reversal of these changes.

Kumar and coworkers[74] investigated the effect of Withania somnifera on oxidative damage induced by chronic constriction injury (CCI) in male Wistar rats. CCI was inflicted by exposing the common sciatic nerve at the middle of the thigh and placing four ligatures 1 mm apart. After ligation, the muscular and skin layers were sutured. The group of rats that underwent this surgery constituted the CCI group. A group of rats that underwent similar surgery without ligation constituted the control group. 21 days after surgery, the CCI group showed increased LPO and nitrite and decreased GSH and CAT in a segment of the sciatic nerve compared to the control group. The CCI group treated with Withania somnifera (100 or 200 mg/kg/day, P.O.) for 21 days after surgery showed a reversal of these changes.

Kyathanahalli and coworkers[75] examined the effect of Withania somnifera roots on diabetes-induced testicular oxidative stress in prepubertal rats. Diabetes was induced in male CFT-Wistar rats by a single intraperitoneal injection of streptozotocin (STZ, 90 mg/kg). Diabetic rats showed increased ROS, LPO and activities of GST and GR in testis cytosol and mitochondria, increased GSH and SOD in testis mitochondria, and decreased total thiol and activities of CAT and GPx in testis cytosol and mitochondria compared to non-diabetic rats. Diabetic rats treated with Withania somnifera for 15 days showed a reversal of these changes.

Kanyaiya and coworkers[76] investigated the antioxidant effect of an aqueous extract of Withania somnifera along with milk in mice. Swiss albino mice were treated with a normal synthetic diet+milk (group A), a normal synthetic diet containing 3% extract (group B), or a normal synthetic diet containing 3% extract+milk (Group C) for 28 days. Groups B and C showed decreased LPO and PC and increased GSH in the liver compared to group A. Group C was more effective than group B. The authors stated that "milk works as good carrier that effectively transfers the phytochemical without affecting its functionality and/or milk constituents interact with the bioactive components of WS thus enhancing its health benefits".

Gopinath and coworkers[77] investigated the effect of a Withania somnifera root extract on chlorpyrifos (o,o-diethyl-3,5,6-trichloro-pyridyl phosphothionate, CPF)-induced oxidative stress in mice. Swiss albino mice treated with CPF for 28 days showed increased LPO and decreased GSH, GR, CAT, SOD and GST in the liver compared to controls. Mice treated with CPF and the extract for 28 days showed a reversal of these changes.

Khalil and coworkers[78] reported that an ethanol extract of Withania somnifera leaves mitigated isoproterenol (ISO)-induced oxidative damage in the rat myocardium. Adult male Wistar rats treated with distilled water (2 ml/kg/day) for 28 days and injected with ISO (85 mg/kg/day) on days 29 and 30 showed increased LPO and decreased SOD, GRx and GPx and GST in heart tissue compared to rats treated with distilled water for 28 days and injected with saline on days 29 and 30. Rats treated with the extract (100 mg/kg/day) for 28 days and injected with ISO on days 29 and 30 showed a reversal of these changes.

Ahmed and coworkers[79] reported that an alcoholic extract of Withania somnifera mitigated the oxidative changes induced by 6-hydroxy-dopamine (6-OHDA) in the rat brain. Male Wistar rats were injected with 2 µl of 6-OHDA (10 µg in 0.1% ascorbic acid-saline) into the right striatum. After 5 weeks, they showed increased LPO and decreased GSH in the substantia nigra as well as decreased GST, GPx, GR, SOD and CAT in the striatum compared to rats that received an ascorbic acid-saline injection into the right striatum. Rats treated with the extract (100-300 mg/kg/day, P.O.) for 21 days followed by a single injection of 6-OHDA showed a reversal of these changes.

References

1   Barry Halliwell "Free radicals and other reactive species in disease" in Encyclopedia of Life Sciences. John Wiley & Sons Ltd, Chichester, 2005. doi:10.1038/npg.els.0003913.
2   Alugoju Phaniendra, Dinesh Babu Jestadi, Latha Periyasamy. Free radicals: properties, sources, targets, and their implication in various diseases. Ind J Clin Biochem (2015) 30 (1): 11-26.
3   Giuseppe Paradies, Giuseppe Petrosillo, Valeria Paradies, Francesca M Ruggiero. Oxidative Stress, mitochondrial bioenergetics and cardiolipin in aging. Free Radical Biology & Medicine (2010) 48: 1286-1295
4   David Hernandez-Garcia, Christopher D Wood, Susana Castro-Obregon, Luis Covarrubias. Reactive oxygen species: a radical role in development. Free Radical Biology & Medicine (2010) 49: 130-143
5   Magdalena L Circu, Tak Yew Aw. Reactive oxygen species, cellular redox systems and apoptosis. Free Radical Biology & Medicine (2010) 48: 749-762
6   V Niviere, M Fontecave. "Biological sources of reduced oxygen species" in Analysis of Free Radicals in Biological Systems. Edited by A E Favier, J Cadet, B Kalyanaraman, M Fontecave. J Lpirre. Birkhauser, Basel 1995.
7   Ron Kohen, Abraham Nyska. Oxidation of biological systems: oxidative stress phenomena, antioxidants, redox reactions and methods for their quantification. Toxicologic Pathology (2002) 30(6): 620-650.
8   Noriko Noguchi, Etsuo Niki. "Chemistry of active oxygen species and antioxidants" in Antioxidant Status. Diet, Nutrition and Health. Edited by Andreas M Papas. CRC Press, Boca Raton, FL, 1998.
9   Kelvin J A Davies. Protein damage and degradation by oxygen radicals. The

Journal of Biological Chemistry (1987) 262 (20): 9895-9901.

10 Kenneth B Beckman, Bruce N Ames, Oxidative decay of DNA. The Journal of Biological Chemistry (1997) 272 (32): 19633-19636.

11 R L Levine, E R Stadtman. Oxidative modifications of protein during aging. Exp Gerontology (2001) 36 (9): 1495-1502.

12 B Palmieri, V Sblendorio. Oxidative stress tests: overview on reliability and use part 1. European Review for Medical and Pharmacological Sciences (2007) 11: 309-342.

13 William R Markesbery, Mark A Lovell. Damage to lipids, proteins, DNA, and RNA in mild cognitive impairment. Archives of Neurology (2007) 64 (7): 954-956.

14 Barry Halliwell, John M C Gutteridge. Free Radicals in Biology and Medicine. Clarendon Press, Oxford, UK, 1999.

15 Helmut Sies. "Oxidative stress: introductory remarks" in Oxidative Stress. Edited by Helmut Sies. Academic Press, London, 1985.

16 Robert A Jacob. The integrated antioxidant system. Nutrition Research (1995) 15 (5): 755-766.

17 Marsden S Blois. Antioxidant determinations by the use of a stable free radical. Nature (1958) 181: 1199-1200.

18 A. Russo, A. A. Izzo, V. Cardile, F. Borrelli and A. Vanella. Indian medicinal plants as antiradicals and DNA cleavage protectors. Phytomedicine (2001) 8 (2): 125-132.

19 Sumathi S, Padma P. R, Gathampari S, and Vidhya S. Free radical scavenging activity of different parts of Withania somnifera. Ancient Science of Life (2007) XXVI (3): 30-34.

20 Prateek Kumar Jain, Veerasamy Ravichandran, Simant Sharma, Ram K. Agrawal. The antioxidant activity of some medicinal plants. Turk J Biol (2008) 32: 197-202.

21 Kanhiya Mahour and Prabhu N. Saxena. In vitro antioxidant status of aqueous extract of Indian Ginseng D. and Panax Ginseng D. Pharmacologyonline (2010) 1: 118-123.

22 Mandal Palash, Ghosal Mitali, Misra Tarun Kumar, Das Abhaya Prasad. Pharmacognostic and free radical scavenging activity in the different parts of Ashwagandha (Withania somnifera (L. Dunal)). Int. J. Drug Dev. & Res (2010) 2 (4): 830-843.

23 Nadia Alam, Monzur Hossain, Md Ibrahim Khalil, Mohammed Moniruzzaman, Siti Amrah Sulaiman and Siew Hua Gan. High catechin concentrations detected in Withania somnifera (ashwagandha) by high performance liquid chromatography analysis. BMC Complementary and Alternative Medicine (2011) 11: 65.

24 Ajay Pal, Mahadeva Naika, Farhath Khanum and Amarinder Singh Bawa. In vitro studies on the antioxidant assay profiling of Withania somnifera L. (Ashwagandha) Dunal root: part 1. Pharmacognosy Journal (2011) 3 (20): 47-55.

25 Rifat-uz-Zaman, Maida Ghaffar, Tehrim Fayyaz, Shumalia Mehdi. In vitro evaluation of total phenolics and antioxidant activities of Withania somnifera, Eclipta prostrata L and Gossypium herbaceum L. J App Pharm (2011) 01(03): 133-144.

26 Nadia Alam, Monzur Hossain, Md Abdul Mottalib, Siti Amrah Sulaiman, Siew Hua Gan, Md Ibrahim Khalil. Methanolic extracts of Withania somnifera leaves, fruits and roots possess antioxidant properties and antibacterial activities. BMC Complementary and Alternative Medicine (2012) 12: 175.

27 Dipankar Chaudhuri, Nikhil Baban Ghate, Rhitajit Sarkar, Nripendranath

Mandal. Phytochemical analysis and evaluation of antioxidant and free radical scavenging activity of Withania somnifera root. Asian Journal of Pharmaceutical and Clinical Research (2012) 5 (4): 193-199.

28 Mohammad Shahriar, Md. Ismail Hossain, Farzana Anwar Sharmin, Sadika Akhter, Md. Aminul Haque and Mohiuddin Ahmed Bhuiyan. In vitro antioxidant and free radical scavenging activity 0f Withania somnifera root. IOSR Journal of Pharmacy (2013) 3 (2): 38-47.

29 Tushar Dhanani, Sonal Shah, N. A. Gajbhiye, Satyanshu Kumar. Effect of extraction methods on yield, phytochemical constituents and antioxidant activity of Withania somnifera. Arabian Journal of Chemistry (2017) 10 (sup1): S 1193 – S1199.

30 G. P. Pathak, Anubhav Khurana, Divesh Sood, Navjot Sharma, Amir, Vineet Sharma. In vitro study of antioxidant activity of Withania somnifera (Ashwagandha) root. American Journal of Pharmtech Research (2013) 3(5): 464-471.

31 Alok Kumar Srivastav, Priyanka Das. Phytochemical extraction and characterization of roots of Withania somnifera for its anti-bacterial, antioxidant, and analgesic activity. International Journal of Innovative Research & Development (2014) 3 (7): 22-33.

32 Lalit Sharma and Arun Sharma. In vitro antioxidant, anti-inflammatory, and antimicrobial activity of hydro-alcoholic extract of roots of Withania somnifera. Journal of Chemical and Pharmaceutical Research (2014) 6 (7): 178-182.

33 Makhija Manju, Gupta Maheshkumar K. In vitro antioxidant activity and HPTLC analysis of Withania somnifera. Journal of Biomedical and Phamaceutical Research (2014) 3 (6): 35-42.

34 Manju Bhaskar and Mena Chintamaneni. Withania somnifera and Ecliptica alba ameliorate oxidative stress induced mitochondrial dysfunction in an animal model of Alzheimer's disease. American Journal of Phytomedicine and Clinical Therapeutics (2014) 2 (1): 140-152.

35 Shakhawat Hossain, Jahidul Islam, Firoj Ahmed, Md. Amjad Hossain, Mohammad Abdul Kalum Siddiki and S. M. Moazzem Hossen. Free radical scavenging activity of six medicinal plants of Bangladesh: a potential source of natural antioxidant. Journal of Applied Pharmacy (2015) 7 (1): 96-104.

36 Sangilimuthu Alagar Yadav, Lukmanul Hakkim. F and R. Sathishkumar. Antioxidant activity of Withania somnifera (L.) Dunal by different solvent extraction methods. Journal of Pharmacy Research (2011) 4 (5): 1428-1430.

37 Ashok Kumar Yadav and Dinesh Chandra Rai. In vitro screening of Ashwagandha root extracts for the maximum functional components. The Pharma Innovation Journal (2018) 7 (2): 12-16.

38 Sunita Panchwat. In vitro free radical scavenging activity of leaves extract of Withania somnifera. Recent Research in Science and Technology (2011) 3 (11): 40-43.

39 Ajay Pal, Mukesh Kumar, Vinod Saharan and Bharat Bhushan. Antioxidant and free radical scavenging activity of Ashwagandha (Withania somnifera L.) leaves. Journal of Global Biosciences (2015) 4 (1): 1127-1137.

40 Ratan Kumar Paul, Homayun Kabir, Uttam Kumar Chowdhury, Md. Saifur Rahman, Md. Faruak Ahmad, Debu Kumar Bhattacharjya. In vitro antioxidant activity of Withania somnifera root. International Journal of Advanced Research in Chemical Sciences (2016) 3 (3): 45-56.

41 E Cadenas, K J A Davies. Mitochondrial free radical generation, oxidative stress and aging. Free Radical Biology & Medicine (2000) 29 (3/4): 222-230.

42 Alicia J Kowaltowski, Nadja C de Souza-Pinto, Roger F Castilho. Anibal E Vercesi. Mitochondria and reactive oxygen species. Free Radical Biology &

Medicine (2009) 47: 333-343.
43 M Valko, C J Rhodes, J Moncol, M Izakovic, M Mazur. Free radicals, metals and antioxidants in oxidative stress-induced cancer. Chemico- Biological Interactions (2006) 160: 1-40.
44 Patel D. S., Shah P. B., Managoli N. B. Evaluation of in vitro anti-oxidant and free radical scavenging activities of Withania somnifera and Aloe vera. Asian J. Pharm. Tech (2012) 2 (4):143-147.
45 T P A Devasagayam, K K Boloor and T Ramasarma. Methods for estimating lipid peroxidation: an analysis of merits and demerits. Indian Journal of Biochemistry & Biophysics (2003) 40: 300-308.
46 Kota V. Ramana, Sanjay Srivastava, and Sharad S. Singhal. Lipid peroxidation products in human health and disease. Oxidative Medicine and Cellular Longevity (2013), Article ID 583438, 3 pages.
47 Ajay Pal, Mahadeva Naika, Farhath Khanum, Amarinder Singh Bawa. In vitro studies on the antioxidant assay profiling of root of Withania somnifera L. (Ashwagandha) Dunal: part 2. Agriculturae Conspectus Scientificus (2012) 77 (2): 95-101.
48 U. Subasini, G. Victor Rajamanickam. Comparative antioxidant evaluation of three Indian cardioprotective medicinal plants in vitro studies. Int J Intg Med Sci (2014) 1 (2); 21-29.
49 Cleva Villanueva, Cecilia Giulivi. Subcellular and cellular locations of nitric oxide synthase isoforms as determinants of health and disease. Free Radicals Biology & Medicine (2010) 49: 307-316.
50 Aline Augusti Boligon, Michel Mansur Machado and Margareth Linde Athayde. Technical evaluation of antioxidant activity. Medicinal Chemistry (2014) 4 (7): 517-522.
51 Sunanda Panda and Anand Kar. Evidence for free radical scavenging activity of Ashwagandha root powder in mice. Indian J Physiol Pharmacol (1997) 41 (4): 424-426.
52 Salil K Bhattacharya, Kalkunte S Satyan & Shibnath Ghosal. Antioxidant activity of glycowithanolides from Withania somnifera. Indian Journal of Experimental Biology (1997) 35: 236-239.
53 A. Bhattacharya, S. Ghosal, S. K. Bhattacharya. Anti-oxidant effect of Withania somnifera glycowithanolides in chronic footshock stress-induced perturbations of oxidative free radical scavenging enzymes and lipid peroxidation in rat frontal cortex and striatum. Journal of Ethnopharmacology (2001) 74: 1-6.
54 Jayant N. Dhuley. Effect of ashwagandha on lipid peroxidation in stress-induced animals. Journal of Ethnopharmacology (1998) 60: 173-178.
55 M S Parihar and Taruna Hemnani. Phenolic antioxidants attenuate hippocampal neuronal cell damage against kainic acid induced excitotoxicity. J. Biosci (2003) 28 (1): 121-128.
56 Salma Khanam and Kshama Devi. Effect of Withania somnifera root extract on lead-induced DNA damage. Journal of Food, Agriculture & Environment (2005) 3 (1): 31-33.
57 Tarique Anwer, Manju Sharma, Krishna Kolappa Pillai and Gyas Khan. Protective effect of Withania somnifera against oxidative stress and pancreatic β-cell damage in type 2 diabetic rats. Acta Poloniae Pharmaceutica- Drug Research (2012) 69 (6): 1095-1101.
58 Pattipati S. Naidu, Amanpreet Singh and Shrinivas K. Kulkarni. Effect of Withania somnifera root extract on resperine-induced orofacial dyskinesia and cognitive dysfunction.Phytother. Res (2006) 20: 140-146.
59 Nishant P. Visavadiya, A. V. R. L. Narasimhacharya. Hypocholesteremic and antioxidant effects of Withania somnifera (Dunal) in hypercholesteremic rats.

Phytomedicine (2007) 14: 136-142.
60 Srinivasagam RajaSankar, Thamilarasan Manivasagam, Sankar Surendran.
    Ashwagandha leaf extract: A potential agent in treating oxidative damage and
    physiological abnormalities seen in a mouse model of Parkinson's disease.
    Neuroscience Letters (2009) 454:11-15.
61 Puneet Kumar and Anil Kumar. Possible neuroprotective effect of Withania
    somnifera root extract against 3-nitropropionic acid-induced behavioral,
    biochemical, and mitochondrial dysfunction in an animal model of
    Huntington's disease. J Med Food (2009) 12 (3): 591-600.
62 Rajangam Udayakumar, Sampth Kasthurirengan, Ayyappan Vasudevan,
    Thankaraj Salammal Mariashibu, Jesudass Joseph Sahaya Rayan, Chang
    Won Choi, Andy Ganapathi, Sei Chang Kim. Antioxidant effect of dietary
    supplement Withania somnifera L. reduce blood glucose levels in alloxan-
    induced diabetic rats. Plants Food Hum Nutr (2010) 65: 91-98.
63 Sadhana Sharma, Veena Sharma, Pracheta, Shatruhan Sharma. Therapeutic
    potential of hydromethanolic root extract of Withania somnifera on
    neurological parameters in Swiss albino mice subjected to lead nitrate.
    International Journal of Current Pharmaceutical Research (2011) 3 (2): 52-56.
64 Smijin Soman, P. K. Korah, S. Jayanarayanan, Jobin Mathew, C. S. Paulose.
    Oxidative stress induced NMDA receptor alteration leads to spatial memory
    deficits in temporal lobe epilepsy: Ameliorative effects of Withania somnifera
    and Withanolide A. Neurochem Res (2012) 37: 1915-1927.
65 Rahul B. Patil, Shreya R. Vora and Meena M. Pillai. Protective effect of
    spermatogenic activity of Withania somnifera (Ashwagandha) in galactose
    stressed mice. Annals of Biological Research. (2012) 3 (8): 4159-4165.
66 Iswar Baitharu, Vishal Jain, Satya Narayan Deep, Kalpana Barhwal Hota,
    Sunil Kumar Hota, Dipti Prasad, Govindasamy Ilavazhagan. Withania
    somnifera root extract ameliorates hypobaric hypoxia induced memory
    impairment in rats. Journal of Ethnopharmacology (2013) 145: 431-441.
67 M. J. Manjunath, Muralidhara. Standardized extract of Withania somnifera
    (Ashwagandha) markedly offsets rotenone-induced locomotor deficits,
    oxidative impairments and neurotoxicity in Drosophila melanogaster. J Food
    Sci Technol (2015) 52 (4): 1971-81.
68 Md. Ejaz Ahmed, Hayate Javed, Mohd Moshahid Khan, Kumar Vaibhav,
    Ajmal Ahmad, Andleeb Khan, Rizwana Tabassum, Farah Islam, Mohammed
    M. Safhi, Fakhrul Islam. Attenuation of oxidative damage-associated cognitive
    decline by Withania somnifera in rat model of streptozotocin-induced
    cognitive impairment. Protoplasma (2013) 250: 1067-1078.
69 Nakuleshwar Dut Jasuja, Preeti Sharma and Suresh C. Joshi. Ameliorating
    effect of Withania somnifera on acephate administered male albino rats.
    African Journal of Pharmacy and Pharmacology (2013) 7 (23): 1554-1559.
70 Tabarak Malik, Devendra Kumar Pandey and Nitu Dogra. Ameliorative
    potential of aqueous root extract of Withania somnifera against paracetamol
    induced liver damage in mice. Pharmacologia (2013) 4(2): 89-94.
71 Mani Chopra, Seema, Vijay Lakshmi Sharma. Protective effect of Withania
    somnifera and vitamin E against cadmium induced toxicity in mice spleen.
    International Journal of Pharmacology & Toxicology Science (2013) 3 (6): 32-
    42.
72 Evan Prince Sabina, Mahaboobkhan Rasool, Mahima Vedi, Dhanalakshmi
    Navaneethan, Meenakshi Ravichander, Poornima Parthasarthy, Sarah Rachel
    Thella. International Journal of Pharmacy and Pharmaceutical Sciences.
    (2013) 5 (2): 648-651.
73 Mahima Vedi, Mahaboobkhan Rasool, Evan Prince Sabina. Amelioration of
    bromobenzene hepatotoxicity by Withania somnifera pretreatment: Role of

mitochondrial oxidative stress. Toxicology Reports (2014) 1: 629-638.

74 Anil Kumar, Seema Meena, Raghavender Pottabathini. Effect of Ashwagandha (Withania somnifera) against chronic constriction injury induced behavioral and biochemical alterations: possible involvement of nitric oxide mechanism. International Journal of Nutrition, Pharmacology, Neurological Diseases (2014) 4 (3): 131-138.

75 Chandrashekara Nagaraj Kythanahalli, Mallayya Jayawanth Manjunath, Muralidhara. Oral supplementation of standardized extract of Withania somnifera protects against diabetes-induced testicular oxidative impairments in prepubertal rats. Protoplasma (2014) 251:1021-1029.

76 Moharkar Kanyaiya, Sawale Pravin Digambar, Sumit Arora, Suman Kapila & R. R. B Singh. In vivo, effect of herb (Withania somnifera) on immunomodulatory and antioxidative potential of milk in mice. Food and Agriculture Immunology (2014) 25 (3): 443-452.

77 Gopinath G, S. Uvarajan, Tamizselvi. A. Chlorpyrifos-induced oxidative stress and tissue damage in the liver of Swiss albino mice: the protective antioxidative role of root extract of Withania somnifera. International Journal for Innovative Research in Science & Technology (2014) 1 (6): 100-104.

78 Md. Ibrahim Khalil, Istiyak Ahmmed, Romana Ahmed, E. M. Tanvir, Rizwana Afroz, Sudip Paul, Siew Hua Gan, and Nadia Alam. Amelioration of isoproterenol-induced oxidative damage in rat myocardium by Withania somnifera leaf extract. BioMed Research International (2015), Article ID 624159, 10 pages.

79 Muzamil Ahmad, Sofiyan Saleem, Abdulla Shafique Ahmad, Mubeen Ahmad Ansari, Seema Yousuf, Md Nasrul Hoda and Fakhrul Islam. Neuroprotective effects of Withania somnifera on 6-hydroxydopamine induced parkinsonism in rats. Human & Experimental Toxicology (2005) 24: 137-147.

3 – Effect on Alzheimer's Disease

3.1 – Introduction

Alzheimer's disease (AD) is a progressive, irreversible neurodegenerative disorder and is the most common form of dementia. It slowly destroys cognitive and behavioral skills and disrupts a person's ability to carry on daily activities. The brains of patients with AD show loss of synapses and neurons as well as two hallmark lesions: extracellular senile plaques and intracellular neurofibrillary tangles (NFTs). The senile plaques mainly contain beta-amyloid peptide. The NFTs are composed of abnormally hyperphosphorylated tau protein. The cause or causes of AD are not completely known. A number of risk factors have been reported which include the following: advanced age, family history and genetic factors, health issues, environmental and lifestyle factors. An estimated 44 million people worldwide have AD or a related form of dementia. In the United States, an estimated 5.5 million people have AD, 5.3 million of whom are 65 years or older. Alzheimer's disease is the sixth leading cause of death in the US[1] and is currently incurable. The drugs that are used offer some symptomatic benefits. FDA approved drugs for managing AD include cholinesterase inhibitors (donepezil, rivastigmine, galantamine) and an NMDA receptor antagonist (memantine). A number of studies have been conducted to examine the effect of Withania somnifera on AD and the results are summarized below.

3.2 – Summary of Results

Tohda and coworkers[2] demonstrated that a methanol extract of Withania somnifera root promoted dendrite formation in SK-N-SH cells. In a subsequent investigation[3], a number of withanolides were isolated from the methanol extract and tested for their neurite outgrowth activities. Human neuroblastoma SH-SY5Y cells were treated with the vehicle or an individual compound (1 µM). After six days, the following compounds were found to induce neurite outgrowth:

- Withanolide A
- (20S,22R)-4β,5β,6α,27-tetrahydroxy-1-oxowitha-2,24-dieno-lide
- Coagulin Q
- Withanoside IV
- Withanoside VI

Another investigation[4] found that in cortical neurons Withanolide A predominantly induced axonal formation, whereas Withanosides IV and VI induced dendritic formation.

Choudhary and coworkers[5] isolated a number of compounds from a methanol extract of Withania somnifera and examined their ability to inhibit the activities of acetylcholinesterase (AChE) and butyryl-cholinesterase (BChE). Acetylthiocholine iodide and butyrylthio-choline chloride were used as substrates to assay AChE and BChE activities respectively. IC_{50} values of compounds that inhibited enzyme activity are presented below (Table 3.1).

Compound	IC_{50} (µM)	
	AChE	BChE
6α,7α-epoxy-3β,5α,20β-trihydroxy-1-oxowitha-24-enolide	Inactive	Inactive
5β,6β-epoxy-4β,17α,27-trihydroxy-1-oxowitha-2,24-dienolide	161.5	Inactive
Withaferin A	84	125
2,3-dihydrowithaferin A	Inactive	500
6α,7α-epoxy-5α,20β-dihydroxy-1-oxowitha-2,24-dienolide	50	Inactive
5β,6β-epoxy-4β-hydroxy-1-oxowitha-2,14,24-trienolide	124	62.5
Galanthamine (positive control)	0.5	8.2
Eserine (positive control)	0.04	0.8

Table 3.1: IC_{50} values of compounds from Withania somnifera and two standard compounds that inhibited AChE and BChE

Kumar and coworkers[6] investigated the kinetics of AChE inhibition by an aqueous extract of Withania somnifera root (WS). WS was found to inhibit the hydrolysis of acetylthiocholine iodide catalyzed by AChE. (IC_{50} = 0.15 mg/ml). The reaction exhibited non-competi-tive inhibition.

Khan and coworkers[7] examined the AChE inhibitory effect of a methanol extract of Withania somnifera and its various fractions. The crude methanol extract was suspended in distilled water and successively partitioned with specific solvents to obtain n-hexane, chloroform, ethyl acetate, n-butanol and aqueous fractions. The hydrolysis of acetylthiocholine iodide catalyzed by AChE in the presence or absence of the extract or each fraction was monitored. The extract and all fractions except n-hexane inhibited AChE activity and the IC_{50} values (µg/ml) are presented below (Table 3.2).

Compound	IC_{50} (µg/ml)
Crude Methanol	76
Chloroform	69
Ethyl acetate	78
n-Butanol	97
Water	111
Galanthamine (positive control)	22.6

Table 3.2: IC_{50} values of different Withania somnifera extracts that inhibited AChE

Kuboyama and coworkers[8] demonstrated that Withanolide A (WLA) induced neuritic regeneration and synaptic reconstruction of cultured neurons damaged by $A\beta_{(25-35)}$ or $A\beta_{(1-42)}$. Rat cortical neurons cultured for 24 hours and treated with $A\beta_{(25-35)}$ or $A\beta_{(1-42)}$ for 4 days showed axonal and dendritic atrophy. Cultured neurons treated with $A\beta_{(25-35)}$ or $A\beta_{(1-42)}$ for 4 days followed by WLA treatment for 4 days showed increased lengths of axons and dendrites. Neurons cultured for 21 days and treated with $A\beta_{(25-35)}$ for 4 days followed by treatment with WLA for 7 days showed a reconstruction of pre- and postsynaptic structures. In vivo studies showed that the injection of $A\beta_{(25-35)}$ into the right ventricle of male ddY mice induced memory impairment and decline of axons, dendrites and synapses in the cerebral cortex and hippocampus. Mice injected with $A\beta_{(25-35)}$ and treated with WLA showed reversal of the changes induced by $A\beta_{(25-35)}$. The authors concluded that "WLA is therefore an important candidate for the therapeutic treatment of neurodegenerative diseases as it is able to reconstruct neuronal networks".

Kumar[9] and coworkers investigated the effects of an aqueous extract of Withania somnifera root (WS) on H_2O_2 and $A\beta_{(1-42)}$ induced cytotoxicity in a differentiated rat pheochromocytoma cell line (dPC12). dPC12 cells are similar to living neurons in the brain. Incubation of dPC12 cells with H_2O_2 (200 μM) for 24 hours reduced cell viability by 50%. Pretreatment of cells with WS protected the cells from H_2O_2 induced cytotoxicity. Similar observations were made in experiments where $A\beta_{(1-42)}$ was used instead of H_2O_2.

Sehgal and coworkers[10] demonstrated that a chloroform-methanol extract of Withania somnifera root (WS) reversed Alzheimer's disease (AD) pathology in AD transgenic mice. Middle-aged male APP/PSI mice, old APP/PSI mice and APPSwInd J20 mice treated with WS for 30 days showed cognitive enhancement and decreased amyloid plaque to varying degrees compared to the corresponding control. WS-treated APP/PSI (old and middle-aged male) mice showed decreased $A\beta_{42}$ in the cortex and hippocampus as well as decreased brain $A\beta_{40}$ and plasma $A\beta_{40/42}$. WS-treated middle-aged female APP/PSI mice showed decreased brain and plasma $A\beta_{42}$. The following observations were made in APP/PSI mice during the 30 day treatment with WS:

- Plaque density decreased in cerebral cortex (CT) after 14 days

- $A\beta_{42}$ monomers decreased in CT after 7 days. Oligomers and total $A\beta_{42/40}$ decreased after 14 days. Plasma $A\beta_{42/40}$ increased between day 7 and 14

- Low-density lipoprotein receptor-related protein (LRP) and LRP mRNA increased in CT after 14 days

- $A\beta$ degrading protease neprilysin (NEP) and NEP mRNA increased only after day 21

- Hepatic LRP, NEP and the plasma soluble form of LRP (SLRP) increased from day 7

The authors stated that "the potent effect of WS in rapidly clearing $A\beta$ is mainly related to its effect in the periphery through increases in the levels of liver LRP and SLRP, indicating that targeting the periphery for $A\beta$ clearance may provide a unique mechanism for rapid elimination of $A\beta$, eventually leading to reversal of behavior deficits in AD transgenic mice".

Kurupati and coworkers[11] evaluated the neuroprotective effects of a methanol-chloroform (3:1) extract of Withania somnifera root (WS) against $A\beta_{(1-42)}$ induced toxicity in human neuronal SK-N-MC cells. The cells were treated with $A\beta_{(1-42)}$ or $A\beta_{(1-42)}$+WS under various experimental conditions. Untreated cells served as a control. Major observations from this study are summarized below (Table 3.3).

Test Assay	SK-N-MC+A$\beta_{(1-42)}$ compared to control	SK-N-MC+A$\beta_{(1-42)}$+WS compared to SK-N-MC+A$\beta_{(1-42)}$
Cell growth	Decreased	Increased
Cell viability	Decreased	Increased
Internalization of A$\beta_{(1-42)}$	Significant	Decreased
LDH release	Increased	Decreased
Spindle density	Decreased	Increased
PPARY levels	Decreased	Increased

Table 3.3: Effects of WS Methanol-Chloroform Extract on A$\beta_{(1-42)}$ Induced Toxicity in SK-N-MC cells

Jayaprakasham and coworkers[12] investigated the effect of Withanamides A (WA) and C (WC) isolated from Withania somnifera fruit on β-amyloid peptide (BAP$_{39-42}$) induced cytotoxicity in PC-12 cells (rat neuronal cells). Incubation of PC-12 cells with BAP inhibited cell growth and increased cell death. Incubation of PC-12 cells with BAP and WA or WC reversed the changes induced by BAP. Electron microscope pictures of MTT crystals deposited by PC-12 cells treated with BAP showed a distorted cell structure and shape, whereas cells treated with BAP+WA showed a regular structure and shape. Molecular modeling studies indicated that WA and WC can bind to the active motif of β amyloid and prevent fibril formation. The authors suggested that "the withanamides present in its fruit can be developed as a prophylaxis and improve the quality of living AD patients".

Vinutha and coworkers[13] reported that a methanol extract of Withania somnifera root inhibited acetylcholinesterase (IC$_{50}$ = 33.8 µg/ml).

Bhatnagar and coworkers[14] examined the effects of Withania somnifera root extract (WS) on NADPH diaphorase (NADPH-d) activity, choline acetyl transferase activity (ChAT), hippocampal serotonin level and serum cortisone level in mice exposed to chronic restraint stress. Adult Swiss albino mice were treated with a normal diet (control group), normal diet+restraint stress (group 1), normal diet+WS+restraint stress (group 2) or normal diet+WS (group 3). The duration of the treatment was 30 days. Group 1 showed an increased number of NADPH-d positive neurons, decreased serotonin, decreased ChAT activity and increased cortisone compared to the control group. Group 2 showed a reversal of these changes. Group 3 and the control group showed similar values. In another investigation, Bhatnagar and coworkers[15] showed that fresh leaf juice of Withania somnifera inhibited acetylcholinesterase and NO synthase activity in the mouse brain.

Jain and coworkers[16] demonstrated that an extract of Withania somnifera root powder reduced the number of stress-induced cell bodies in the hippocampal subregions of female albino rats.

References

1   Alzheimer's Disease Statistics, Alzheimer's News Today. https://alzheimersnewstoday.com/alzheimers-disease-statistics/
2   Tohda C, Kuboyama T, Komatsu K. Dendrite extension by methanol extract of Ashwagandha (roots of Withania somnifera) in SK-N-SH cells. Neuroreport (2000) 11 (9): 1981-5.
3   Jing Zhao, Norio Nakamura, Masao Hattori, Tomoharu Kuboyama, Chihiro Tohda, and Katsuko Komatsu. Withanolide derivatives from the roots of Withania somnifera and their neurite outgrowth activities. Chem Pharm Bull (2002) 50 (6): 760-765.
4   Tomoharu Kuboyama, Chihiro Tohda, Jing Zhao, Norio Nakamura, Masao Hattori and Katsuko Komatsu. Axon- or dendrite-predominant outgrowth induced by constituents from Ashwagandha. Neurochemistry (2002) 13(14): 1715-1720.
5   Muhammad Iqbal Choudhary, Sammer Yousuf, Sarfraz Ahmad Nawaz, Shakil Ahmed, and Atta-Ur- Rahman. Cholinesterase inhibiting withanolides from Withania somnifera. Chem Pharm Bull (2004) 52 (11): 1358-1361.
6   Suresh Kumar, Christopher John Seal and Edward Jonathan Okello. Kinetics of acetylcholinesterase inhibition by an aqueous extract of Withania somnifera roots. IJSPR (2011) 2(5): 1188-1192.
7   Haroon Khan, Shafiq Ahmad Tariq, Murad Ali Khan, Inayat-Ur-Rehman, Rukhsana Ghaffar and Saifullah. Cholinesterase and lipoxygenase inhibition of whole plant of Withania somnifera. African Journal of Pharamacy and Pharmacology (2011) 5(20): 2272-2275.
8   Tomoharu Kuboyama, Chihiro Tohda and Katsuko Komatsu. Neuritic regeneration and synaptic reconstruction induced by withanolide A. British Journal of Pharmacology (2005) 144:961-971.
9   Kumar S, Seal CJ, Howes M-JR, Kite GC, Okello EJ. Invitro protective effects of Withania somnifera (L) Dunal root extract against hydrogen peroxide and β-amyloid (1-42) induced cytotoxicity in differentiated PC12 cells. Phytotherpy Research (2010) 24 (10): 1567-74.
10 Neha Sehgal, Alok Gupta, Rupanagudi Khader Valli, Shanker Datt Joshi, Jessica T. Mills, Edith Hamel, Pankaj Khanna, Subhash Chand Jain, Suman S. Thakur, and Vijayalakshmi Ravindranath. Withania somnifera reverses Alzheimer's disease pathology by enhancing low-density lipoprotein receptor-related protein in liver. PNAS (2012) 109 (9): 3510-3515.
11 Kesava Rao Venkata Kurapati, Venkata Subbarao Atluri, Thangavel Samikkannu, Madhavan P. N. Nair. Ashwagandha (Withania somnifera)

reverses β-amyloid1-42 induced toxicity in human neuronal cells: Implications in HIV-associated neurocognitive disorders (HAND). PLOS ONE (2013) 8 (10): e77624.

12 Bolleddula Jayaprakasam, Kaillathe Padmanabhan and Muraleedharan G. Nair. Withanolides in Withania somnifera fruit protect PC-12 cells from β-amyloid responsible for Alzheimer's disease. Phytother Res (2010) 24: 859-863.

13 B. Vinutha, D. Prashanth, K. Salma, S. L. Sreeja, D. Pratiti, R. Padmaja, S. Radhika, A. Amit, K. Venkateshwarlu, M. Deepak. Screening of selected Indian medicinal plants for acetylcholinesterase inhibitory activity. Journal of Ethnopharmacology (2007) 109: 359-363.

14 Maheep Bhatnagar, Durgesh Sharma, Mahendra Salvi. Neuroprotectve effects of Withania somnifera Dunal: A possible mechanism. Neurochem Res (2009) 34: 1975-1983.

15 M. Bhatnagar, P. Suhalka, P. Sukhawal, A. Jain, and D. Sharma. Inhibition of acetylcholinesterase and NO synthase activity in the mice brain: Effect of Withania somnifera leaf juice. Neurophysiology (2012) 44 (4): 301-308.

16 Sushma Jain, Sunil Dutt Shukla, Kanika Sharma and Maheep Bhatnagar. Neuroprotective effects of Withania sonifera Dunn. in hippocampal subregions of female albino rat. Phytother Res (2001) 15: 544-548.

4 – Effects on Parkinson's and Huntington's Diseases

4.1 – Parkinson's Disease

Parkinson's disease (PD) is a chronic, progressive neurological disorder. It is the second most common neurodegenerative disorder after Alzheimer's Disease. PD develops with the progressive loss of dopamine-producing neurons in the substantia nigra region of the brain. Dopamine plays an important role in many processes including voluntary movements, behavior, cognition and mood. The primary motor symptoms of PD are tremors, rigidity, bradykinesia (slowness of motion) and postural instability. Non-motor symptoms include cognitive impairment, depression, anxiety, sleep disturbance and psychosis[1]. As the disease progresses, individuals experience difficulty in walking, talking and performing tasks. The exact cause of PD is unknown but several risk factors have been identified. An estimated 7-10 million people worldwide and 1 million in the U.S. have PD[2]. Currently, there is no cure for PD, but drugs are available to control the symptoms. These drugs include levodopa (L-Dopa), dopamine agonists, inhibitors of enzymes that inactivate dopamine, anticholinergics and antiviral drugs. A number of investigators have examined the effect of Withania somnifera in animal models of Parkinson's disease and the results are summarized below.

Ahmad and coworkers[3] examined the neuroprotective effects of an ethanol extract of Withania somnifera (WS) on 6-hydroxydopamine (6-OHDA)-induced parkinsonism in rats. Male Wistar rats injected with 6-OHDA dissolved in ascorbic acid-saline solution into the right striatum showed the following neurobehavioral and biochemical changes compared to the sham group (injected with only ascorbic acid-saline solution):

- neurobehavioral impairment (elevation in rotations, reduced locomotor time and decreased muscular coordination)
- increased LPO and decreased GSH (substantia nigra)

- decreased GST, GPx, GR, SOD, CAT, DA, DOPAC and HVA (striatum)
- increased dopaminergic D_2 receptor binding in synaptic membrane fractions prepared from the right striatum
- decreased expression of tyrosine hydroxylase in the ipsilateral striatum

Rats treated with WS (100, 200 or 300 mg/kg/day) for 21 days before the administration of 6-ODHA showed a reversal of these changes. The authors concluded that "the study demonstrates that the extract of W. Somnifera may be helpful in protecting the neuronal injury in Parkinson's disease".

Raja Sankar and coworkers[4] investigated the effect of a Withania somnifera root extract on parkinsonism in mice induced by 1-methyl-4-phenyl-1,2,3,6-tetrahydropyridine (MPTP). Male albino mice treated with MPTP (20 mg/kg/day, i.p.) for 4 days showed neurobehavioral impairments (reduced retention time in the rotarod test, reduced hang time in the hang test and decreased stride length) as well as increased LPO, SOD and CAT in the midbrain compared to controls. Mice treated with MPTP (20 mg/kg/day, i.p.) for 4 days followed by WS (100 mg/kg/day, P.O.) for 28 days showed a reversal of these changes. A similar study[5] showed that treating male albino mice with MPTP (20 mg/kg/day, i.p.) for 4 days increased LPO and decreased DA, DOPAC, HVA, GSH and GPx in the striatum compared to controls. Treating mice with MPTP for 4 days followed by WS (100 mg/kg/day, P.O.) for 28 days reversed these changes. The authors concluded that "These data suggest that WS is a potential drug in treating catecholamines, oxidative damage and physiological abnormalities seen in the PD mouse".

Raja Sankar and coworkers[6] also examined the effect of a Withania somnifera leaf extract (WS) on oxidative damage and physiological abnormalities in mice induced by MPTP. Male Swiss albino mice treated with MPTP (20 mg/kg/day, i.p.) for four days showed increased LPO, CAT and SOD, decreased GSH and GPx in the midbrain and striatum, and impaired motor functions. Mice treated with WS (100 mg/kg/day, P.O.) for 3 days followed by WS+MPTP for another four days showed a reversal of the changes induced by MPTP.

Prakash and coworkers[7] examined the neuroprotective role of an ethanol extract of Withania somnifera roots (WS) on a maneb-paraquat (MB-PQ)-induced model of parkinsonism. MB is a fungicide and PQ is a herbicide. They are known to induce oxidative stress and cause neurotoxicity. They act synergistically when given together. Swiss albino mice treated with MB (30 mg/kg, i.p.)+PQ (10 mg/kg, i.p.) twice weekly for 3, 6 and 9 weeks showed the following changes compared to the control group:

- impaired motor behavior

- increased LPO and nitrite and decreased CAT in nigrostriatal tissue

- reduced tyrosine hydroxylase (TH) immunoreactivity in the substantia nigra (TH is a rate-limiting enzyme in the dopamine synthesis pathway)

Mice treated with MB+PQ along with WS (100 mg/kg/day, P.O.) showed a reversal of the changes induced by MB+PQ. The authors concluded that "our results clearly indicate the usefulness of WS root extract in providing protection against MB-PQ induced nigrostriatal dopaminergic neurodegeneration and marked improvement in the behavioral, anatomical and biochemical deformities". Another study[8] demonstrated that WS treatment provides protection in MB-PQ-induced parkinsonism by modulating oxidative stress and apoptotic machinery. Prakash and coworkers[9] also demonstrated a synergistic neuroprotective effect of Mucuna pruriens (MP) and Withania somnifera (WS) in a paraquat-induced mouse model of parkinsonism. The authors suggested that "MP and WS may provide a platform for future drug discoveries and novel treatment strategies for PD".

4.2 – Huntington's Disease (HD)

Huntington's disease is a hereditary, progressive, neurodegenerative disorder. It is characterized by involuntary movements, cognitive deficits and psychiatric/behavioral changes. HD is caused by a mutation in the HTT gene, which is located on chromosome 4 and codes for the protein huntingtin. The mutated gene produces huntingtin with many more CAG (cytosine-adenine-guanine) units than the huntingtin produced by the normal gene (less than 27 CAG repeats). The altered form of huntingtin leads to the death of neurons in specific parts of the brain, and individuals with CAG repeats of 36 or more develop the disease[10]. HD is inherited in an autosomal dominant manner. Children of mutated HTT carriers have a 50% chance of inheriting the disease.

There are two forms of HD: early-onset (symptoms appear in childhood or teens) and adult-onset (symptoms manifest in the mid-30s or 40s). Currently, there is no cure for HD, but a number of treatments are available to manage the symptoms. A few studies have examined the effect of Withania somnifera on symptoms of Huntington's disease using animal models. The results are summarized below.

Kumar and Kumar[11] examined the effect of a Withania somnifera root extract (WS) on behavioral and biochemical changes induced by 3-nitropropionic acid (3-NP) in rats. 3-NP administration produces HD-like symptoms in rats. Male Wistar rats treated with 3-NP (10 mg/kg, i.p.) for 14 days showed the following changes compared to controls:

- decreased rearing scores, decreased performance on the rotarod test and decreased hind limb retraction in the limb withdrawal test

- decreased enzyme complexes I, II and III in whole brain mitochondria

- increased LPO, nitrite levels and LDH and decreased SOD and CAT in the striatum and cortex

Treating rats with WS (100 or 200 mg /kg, P.O.) one hour before the administration of 3-NP reversed these changes. The authors concluded that "These findings suggest that neuroprotective actions of W. somnifera are mediated via its antioxidant activity. However, further studies are required to elucidate the molecular mechanisms involved in order to support the clinical use of the plant extract as a therapeutic agent for the treatment of HD".

Venkataramaniah and Praba[12] examined the effect of an ethanol extract of Withania somnifera (WS) and Withanolide D (WD) in rats exhibiting HD-like symptoms induced by kainic acid. Adult male Sprague Dawly rats injected with kainic acid into the striatum exhibited choreiform movements in both the head region and limbs. The animals were also unable to stay on a rotarod until the end of the test (180 sec). The animals in the sham group as well as animals treated with WS (125 mg/kg) or WD (100 mg/kg) for 10 days and injected with kainic acid showed no choreiform movements and stayed on the rotarod till the end of the test. The authors concluded that "by taking these herbal drugs on a daily basis we can prevent the occurrence of HD as these drugs are very good in neuroprotection". In a similar investigation, Praba and coworkers[13] showed that rats treated with WS or WD for 10 days and injected with kainic acid performed better on the narrow beam test compared with animals injected with kainic acid without WS or WD pretreatment.

References

1   George DeMaagd and Ashok Philip. Parkinson's disease and its management. Part 1: Disease entity, risk factors, Pathophysiology, Clinical presentation, and Diagnosis. P & T (2015) 40 (8): 504-532.
2   Parkinson's Disease Statistics. Parkinson's News Today. https://parkinsonsnewstoday.com/parkinsons-disease-statistics/
3   Muzamil Ahmad, Sofiyan Saleem, Abdullah Shafique Ahmad, Mubeen Ahmad Ansari, Seema Yousuf, Md Nasrul Hoda and Fakhrul Islam. Neuroprotective effects of Withania somnifera on 6-hydroxydopamine induced parkinsonism in rats. Human and Experimental Toxicology (2005) 24: 137-147.
4   Srinivasagam Raja Sankar, Thamilarasan Manivasagam, Arumugam Krishnamurti and Manickam Ramanathan. The neuroprotective effect of Withania somnifera root extract in MPTP-intoxicated mice: an analysis of behavioral and biochemical variables. Cellular & Molecular Biology Letters (2007) 12: 473-481.
5   Srinivasagam Raja Sankar, Thamilarasan Manivasagam, Venkatachalam Sankar, Seppan Prakash, Rathinasamy Muthusamy, Arumugam Krishnamurti, Sankar Surendran. Withania somnifera root extract improves catecholamines and physiological abnormalities seen in a Parkinson's disease model mouse. Journal of Ethnopharmacology (2009) 125 (3): 369-373.
6   Srinivasagam Raja Sankar, Thamilarasan Manivasagam, Sankar Surendran. Ashwagandha leaf extract: A potential agent in treating oxidative damage and physiological abnormalities seen in a mouse model of Parkinson's disease. Neuroscience Letters (2009) 454: 11-15.
7   Jay Prakash, Satyndra Kumar Yadav, Shikha Chohan, Surya Pratap Singh. Neuroprotective role of Withania somnifera root in maneb-paraquat induced mouse model of parkinsonism. Neurochemical Research (2013) 38 (5): 972-80.
8   Jay Prakash, Shikha Chouhan, Satyndra Kumar Yadav, Susan Westfall, Sachchida Nand Rai, Surya Pratap Singh. Withania somnifera alleviates parkinsonian phenotypes by inhibiting apoptotic pathways in dopaminergic neurons. Neurochem Res (2014) 39: 2527-2536.
9   Jay Prakash, Satyndra Kumar Yadav, Shikha Chouhan, Satya Prakash, Surya Pratap Singh. Synergistic effect of Mucuna pruriens and Withania somnifera in a paraquat induced Parkinsonian mouse model. Advances in Bioscience and Biotechnology (2013) 4: 1-9.
10 S. Mahalingam and L. M. Levy. Genetics of Huntington disease. American Journal of Neuroradiology (2014) 36 (6): 1070-1072.
11 Puneet Kumar and Anil Kumar. Possible neuroprotective effect of Withania somnifera root extract against 3-nitropropionic acid-induced behavioral, biochemical, and mitochondrial dysfunction in an animal model of Huntington's disease. Journal of Medicinal Food (2009) 12 (3): 591-600.
12 C. Venkataramaniah, A. Mary Antony Praba. A study on the behavior of Huntington's chorea rat models on rotarod: treated with Withanolide A and ethanolic extract of Withania somnifera. Int J Anat Res (2015) 3 (4): 1510-1514.
13 Mary Antony Praba, C. Venkataramaniah and G. Kavitha. Neuroprotection of ethanolic extract of Withania somnifera and Withanolide A in motor co-ordination on experimental Huntington's rat model. International Journal of Pharmaceutical Sciences and Research (2018) 9 (11): 4800-4804.

5 – Anxiolytic, Antidepressant and Antistress Activities

5.1 – Introduction

Anxiety is an emotion that is a normal part of life. It is generally a feeling of nervousness, worry and fear. These feelings come and go without significantly affecting daily activities. However, when a person experiences a high level of anxiety that persists for a long time, it becomes a medical disorder known as anxiety disorder. According to the World Health Organization, an estimated 264 million people worldwide[1] and 40 million adults in the US[2] suffer from anxiety disorder. Anxiety disorders are generally treated with psychotherapy, medication or both.

Depression is a mood disorder. Typically, people will experience feelings like frustration, helplessness and sadness for relatively short periods. However, if the symptoms persist for longer periods, they can lead to a mental disorder (depressive disorder). Symptoms of depressive disorder include sadness, loss of pleasure, inability to concentrate, fatigue, disturbed sleep or appetite, feelings of guilt and low self-worth, and thoughts of suicide. According to the World Health Organization, an estimated 300 million people worldwide[1] and 19 million teens and adults in the US[3] suffer from depressive disorder. Depressive disorders are generally treated with psychotherapy, medication or both. Anxiety and depression can occur together.

Most people experience stress at one time or another. It is a natural reaction to change or challenge. The same situation may not affect different people the same way. What one feels as a minor inconvenience may be felt as life-threatening by another. It is difficult to define stress precisely. Hans Selye, a pioneer in stress research, defined stress as the nonspecific response of the body to any demand[4]. Recently, Koolhaas and coworkers[5] have proposed that the term stress should be restricted to conditions where an environmental demand exceeds the natural regulatory capacity of an organism, particularly situations that include unpredictability and uncontrollability. Small amounts of stress for a short duration may not be harmful but chronic stress may lead to serious health problems. When a situation is perceived as a threat, it triggers a series of responses from several physiological systems. The sympathetic-adrenal-medullary (SAM) system and the hypothalamic-pituitary-adrenal (HPA) axis are considered to be the two most important pathways that mediate the stress response[6]. Activation of these pathways releases glucocorticoids and catecholamines into the bloodstream[7]. These hormones enable the body to effectively respond and adapt to demanding internal and external stimuli. Prolonged and repeated activation of the SAM and HPA systems can increase the risk for physical and psychiatric disorders[8].

A number of studies have been conducted to examine the anxiolytic, antidepressant and antistress activities of Withania somnifera and the results are summarized below.

5.2 – Summary of Results

Bhattacharya and coworkers[9] examined the anxiolytic and antidepressant effects of Withania somnifera glycowithanolides (WSG) in rats. Charles Foster male rats were treated with WSG (20 or 50 mg/kg/day, P.O.) for 5 days. Anxiolytic effects were evaluated by the elevated plus maze (EPM), social interaction (SI), and novelty suppressed feeding latency (NSFL) tests. Antidepressant effects were assessed by the swim stress-induced behavioral despair (SSIBD), learned helplessness (LH), and rotarod (RR) tests. The following observations were made in the WSG-treated group compared to controls, indicating anxiolytic and antidepressant effects of WSG.

Observations for anxiolytic effects:

- Increased number of entries and time spent on open arms (EPM)

- Increased time spent in social interactions (SI)

- Decreased latency to feed in the test chamber (NSFL)

Observations for antidepressant effects:

- Decreased duration of immobility (SSIBD)

- Decreased escape failures and increased avoidance response (LH)

The anxiolytic effects of WSG were comparable to lorazepam (anxiolytic drug). The antidepressant effects were comparable to imipramine (antidepressant drug). The authors concluded that "the present investigation supports the observations made with WS extracts and the use of these extracts in Ayurveda for stabilization of disturbed mood".

Gupta and Rana[10] reported that an alcohol extract of Withania somnifera root (WS) mitigated alcohol withdrawal anxiety. Rats deprived of alcohol for 72 hours after receiving it for 15 days exhibited alcohol withdrawal anxiety. Withdrawal anxiety was reduced by treatment with WS (200 or 500 mg/kg, P.O.).

Khan and Ghosh[11] demonstrated the anxiolytic activity of Withaferin A (WA) in rats subjected to restrained stress. Male Wistar rats subjected to restrained stress and then treated with WA (10-40 mg/kg, i.p.) or diazepam (0.3, 1.0, or 3.0 mg/kg, i.p.) showed increased open arm exploration time in the elevated plus maze compared to controls. The effect of WA (40 mg) was comparable to diazepam (1mg). Subchronic administration of diazepam (1mg/kg, i.p.) for 6 days produced tolerance, whereas subchronic administration of WA (40 mg/kg, i.p.) enhanced anxiolytic efficacy. The authors stated that WA "may represent a novel class of anti-anxiety agents which may produce continued anxiolytic efficacy following repeated administration, without tolerance liability".

Afsal and coworkers[12] examined the antidepressant activity of EPIC-QTAB, an Ayurvedic polyherbal formulation of Ashwagandha in mice. Antidepressant activity was assessed by the forced swim test (FST) and tail suspension test (TST). Mice treated with EPIC-QTAB showed a significant decrease in immobility time compared to controls.

Shah and coworkers[13] examined the antidepressant activity of Withania somnifera root extract (WS) in mice and its interactions with the conventional antidepressants imipramine (IMP) and fluoxetine (FLT). The forced swim test was used to evaluate antidepressant activity. Albino mice treated with WS (25-100 mg/kg, i.p.), IMP (2.5-10 mg/kg, i.p.) or FLT (2.5-10 mg/kg, i.p.) showed a dose-dependent decrease in mean immobility time (MIT) compared to controls. The effect of WS (100 mg) was comparable to IMP (10 mg) and FLT (10 mg). Lower doses of WS (<50 mg), IMP (<5 mg) and FLT (<5 mg) did not produce a statistically significant reduction in MIT. However, WS (37.5 mg/kg) + IMP (2.5 mg/kg) or WS (37.5 mg/kg) + FLT (2.5 mg/kg) showed a statistically significant reduction in MIT, indicating that WS enhances the effects of IMP and FLT.

Maity and coworkers[14] evaluated the antidepressant effect of Withania somnifera (WS) compared to Bacopa monniera (BM) and
imipramine (IMP). The forced swim and learned helplessness tests
were used to evaluate antidepressant activity. Albino rats treated with
WS (50-150 mg/kg/day, P.O.), BM (20-80 mg/kg/day, P.O.) or IMP
(16-64 mg/kg/day, P.O.) for 14 days showed dose-dependent antidepressant activity in both the forced swim test and learned helplessness test. Also, rats treated with WS (50 mg/kg/day, P.O.) + IMP (16
mg/kg/day, P.O.) or BM (20 mg/kg/day, P.O.) + IMP (16 mg/kg/
day, P.O.) showed significant antidepressant activity. The antidepressant effect decreased in the following order:

- Forced swim: IMP (16 mg) + WS (50 mg) > WS (150 mg) >
  IMP (64 mg) > IMP (16 mg) + BM (20 mg) > BM (80 mg)

- Learned helplessness: IMP (16 mg) + WS (50 mg) > IMP
  (64 mg) > WS (150 mg) > IMP (16 mg) + BM (20 mg) > BM
  (80 mg)

Jayanthi and coworkers[15] examined the antidepressant activity of
ashwagandha ghrutha (AGG), a special formulation of Withania
somnifera. AGG was prepared by boiling a mixture of Withania
somnifera, ghee (clarified butter) and water. After evaporating water,
the ghee portion was filtered and used. Antidepressant activity was
evaluated using the forced swim test (FST), tail suspension test
(TST) and anti-reserpine test (ART). Imipramine (IMP) was also
studied for comparison. Swiss albino mice were divided into several
groups and treated as follows:

Acute study (AS)	Chronic study (CS)
1AS: Normal saline	1CS: 7 days normal saline
2AS: single dose of IMP (15 mg/kg)	2CS: 7 days IMP (15 mg/kg/day)
3AS: single dose of AGG (40 mg/kg)	3CS: 7 days AGG (40 mg/kg/day)
4AS: IMP+AGG	4CS: 7 days IMP+AGG

Each group was subjected to FST and TST after the treatment.
Groups 2, 3 and 4 showed a decreased immobility period compared
to group 1. Chronic treatment produced a greater effect. IMP+AGG
was more effective than IMP or AGG alone. Antidepressant activity
was evaluated with the antireserpine test by a similar procedure with
minor modifications. After the administration of saline, IMP, AGG,
or IMP+AGG, reserpine (2.5 mg/kg, i.p.) was administered. Groups
2, 3 and 4 showed a reduction of reserpine-induced ptosis, catatonia
and sedation compared to group 1. The authors concluded that "In
the light of observations made it may be envisaged that Withania
somnifera can be used as a potential adjuvant in the treatment of
depressive disorders".

Katare and coworkers[16] evaluated the anxiolytic effect of hydroalcoholic extracts of W. somnifera root, C. asiatica whole plant, O. sanctum leaves and a polyherbal formulation containing all three in equal amounts. No anxiolytic effect was observed when Swiss albino mice were treated with the herbs alone. However, the polyherbal formulation showed a significant anxiolytic effect. The authors concluded that the "formulation showed anxiolytic activity and this may be due to synergism between Centella asiatica, Withania somnifera and Ocium sanctum".

Makawana and coworkers[17] reported that Withania somnifera, Berberis aristata and Mucuna pruriens work synergistically to enhance antidepressant activity in Swiss albino mice.

Mirzaei and coworkers[18] demonstrated the anxiolytic activity of an ethanol extract of Withania somnifera root (WS) in rats. Anxiety was evaluated using the elevated plus maze test. Adult male Wistar rats treated with WS (25-150 mg/kg, i.p.) showed a dose-dependent increase in time spent and number of entries into the open arm compared to controls. The dose of 75 mg/kg was found to be optimal. The effect of WS (75 mg/kg) was comparable to the effect of diazepam (1 mg/kg, i.p.).

Bharathi and coworkers[19] reported the antidepressant activity of an aqueous extract of Withania somnifera root (AEWS) in mice. Swiss albino mice treated with AEWS (30, 40 or 50 mg/kg) showed dose-dependent decreases in immobility period (forced swim test) compared to controls. The effect of AEWS (50 mg/kg) was comparable to imipramine (15 mg/kg).

Gopala Krishna and coworkers[20] evaluated the anxiolytic activity of NR-ANX-C, a polyherbal formulation containing Withania somnifera, Ocimum sanctum, Camellia sinensis and Shilajit. In the acute study, male Wistar rats were treated with the vehicle (control), diazepam (0.5 or 1 mg/kg) or NR-ANX-C (5-20 mg/kg) and an hour later were subjected to the elevated plus maze (EPM) or bright and dark arena (BDA) tests. In the EPM test, both diazepam- and NR-ANX-C-treated rats showed a dose-dependent increase in the duration of time spent in the open arms and number of entries into the open arm compared to controls. The effect of NR-ANX-C (10 mg/kg) was comparable to diazepam. In the BDA test, both diazepam- and NR-NX-C-treated rats showed an increase in the duration of time spent and the number of entries into the light chamber compared to controls. The effect of NR-NX-C (10 mg/kg) was comparable to diazepam (1mg). In the chronic study, rats were treated with the vehicle, diazepam (0.5 or 1 mg/kg) or NR-ANX-C (5-20 mg/kg) for 10 days and subjected to the EPM or BDA tests. Results were similar to those obtained in the acute study. A later investigation[21] demonstrated the anxiolytic activity of NR-ANX-C in rats experiencing ethanol withdrawal anxiety. The effect of NR-ANX-C (40 mg/kg) was comparable to the standard drug alprazolam (0.08 mg/kg).

Kumar and Kiran[22] demonstrated the anxiolytic activity of mentat, a polyherbal formulation containing Withania somnifera. Adult Wistar albino rats treated with mentat (300 or 600 mg/kg, P.O.), twice daily for 7 days showed an increased duration of time spent in the open arm and number of entries to the open arm in the elevated plus maze test compared to controls. The effect of mentat (600 mg) was comparable to the anxiolytic drug alprazolam (0.25 mg).

Kulkarni and coworkers[23,24] reported that mentat suppressed the development of morphine tolerance and reversed diazepam-induced hyperactivity in mice. In another investigation, Kulkarni and Ninan[25] showed that Withania somnifera root extract inhibited morphine tolerance and dependence.

Kaurav and coworkers[26] investigated the effects of methanolic (MEWS) and aqueous (AEWS) extracts of Withania somnifera root on obsessive compulsive disorder (OCD) in mice. Swiss albino mice treated with AEWS (25-100 mg/kg), MEWS (25-100 mg/kg) or fluoxetine (10 or 15 mg/kg) showed a reduction in the number of marbles buried compared to controls (marble burying behavior test). Mice treated with AEWS (100 mg/kg) or MEWS (100 mg/kg) showed decreased locomotor activity (assessed by actophotometer). Mice treated with AEWS (10 mg/kg), MEWS (10 mg/kg) or fluoxetine (5 mg/kg) showed no effect on marble-burying behavior compared to controls. However, mice treated with AEWS (10 mg/kg) + fluoxetine (5 mg/kg) or MEWS (10 mg/kg) + fluoxetine (5 mg/kg) showed a reduced number of marbles buried. The authors concluded that "W. extract is effective in treating obsessive compulsive disorder".

Singh and coworkers[27] examined the antistress effect of an alcohol extract of Withania somnifera defatted seeds (WS) in mice and rats subjected to stress. Mice treated with WS (100 mg/kg, i.p.) and subjected to the swimming endurance test showed an increase in the duration of swimming time and a decrease in ascorbic acid and cortisol in the adrenals compared to controls. Adult albino rats treated with WS (100 mg/kg, i.p.) and subjected to cold restraint stress for 2 hours, restraint stress for 18 hours, or treated with aspirin (200 mg/kg, i.p.) showed a decreased ulcer index compared to animals not treated with WS and subjected to stress or treated with aspirin. Mice treated with graded doses of WS (PO) and milk (0.1 ml, SC) showed a reduction of leukocytes compared to mice treated with milk only.

Bhattacharya and coworkers[28] found that a methanol-water extract of Withania somnifera (SG-1) and an equimolar combination of sitoin-dosides VII and VIII (SG-2) mitigated the adverse effects induced by a variety of acute stress paradigms. In rats, SG-1 and SG-2 diminished pentylenetetrazole-induced defecation and urination, restraint stress-induced gastric ulcers, autoanalgesia, morphine thermic response, and depletion of adrenal ascobic acid and corticosterone. In mice, SG-1 and SG-2 attenuated forced swimming-induced immobility and morphine-induced toxicity in overcrowded and tactile-stressed mice. In another study, Bhattacharya and Muruganandam[29] demonstrated the adaptogenic activity of an aqueous-ethanol (1:1) extract of Withania somnifera root (WS) using a rat model of chronic stress. Adult male Wistar rats subjected to mild, unpredictable shocks once daily for 21 days showed gastric ulceration, hyperglycemia and glucose intolerance, behavioral depression, sexual dysfunction, cognitive impairment, immunosuppression and increased plasma corticosterone levels. Treatment with WS (25 and 50 mg/kg/day, P.O.) one hour before the electric shock diminished the effects of the shock.

Archana and Namasivayam[30] evaluated the antistress effect of Withania somnifera root powder (WSR) in rats subjected to cold swimming stress. Adult Wistar rats subjected to cold swimming stress showed increased plasma corticosterone compared to controls. Rats treated with an aqueous suspension of WSR (100 mg/kg/day, via gastric intubation) for 7 days showed an increased swimming time and decreased plasma corticosterone compared to rats subjected to swimming stress without prior treatment with WSR.

Singh and coworkers[31] investigated the adaptogenic activity of a withanolide-free aqueous fraction of Withania somnifera root (BF) against a variety of stressors in mice/rats. Swiss albino mice were used to study the effect of BF on hypoxia time, swimming performance time and fatigue. Charles Foster rats were used to study the effect on swimming-induced gastric ulceration, immobilization-induced autoanalgesia and swimming-induced hypothermia. Mice/rats were treated with the vehicle (P.O.) or BF (12.5-100 mg/kg/day, P.O.) for 15 days and subjected to stress one hour after the last treatment. The animals treated with BF showed a dose-dependent increase in hypoxia time and swimming performance along with decreased fatigue, autoanalgesia, ulcerogenic indices and inhibition of hypothermia compared to mice/rats treated with vehicle and subjected to stress. In another investigation, Singh and coworkers[32] examined the antistress activity of BF in mice/rats against chemical and physical stressors. Major observations from this investigation are summarized below:

- Rats treated with BF (12.5-100 mg/kg, P.O.) showed a dose-dependent inhibition of pedal edema induced by carrageenan. BF (100 mg) was more effective than phenylbutazone (50 mg).

- Treating mice with BF (12.5-100 mg/kg/day, P.O.) for 7 days post-immunization with SRBC showed a significant influence on primary antibody synthesis. BF (100 mg) was more effective than levamisole (2.5 mg/kg).

- Treatment of rats with BF (12.5-100 mg/kg/day, P.O.) for 14 days mitigated the hepatic injury induced by CCl_4 stress or swimming stress. Normal rats subjected to CCl_4 or swimming stress showed increased serum SGPT, SGOT, ALP and triglycerides as well as increased hepatic glycogen and LPO compared to controls. Rats treated with BF and subjected to stress showed a reversal of these changes. The authors concluded that "Our results suggest that oral administration of BF is capable of increasing the capacity to tolerate non-specific stress in experimental animals as evident from the restoration of a large number of parameters studied and does not interfere with the normal physiological conditions of the body".

Jain and coworkers[33] examined the antistress activity of Withania somnifera extracts in mice. The extracts were prepared by conventional methods. Antistress activity was assessed by the elevated plus maze test. Treatment of mice with an extract prepared by maceration using water, a hydroalcoholic extract prepared by soxhlet, or a hydroalcoholic extract prepared by maceration increased the duration of stay in the open arms compared to controls, indicating antistress activity.

Anju[34] evaluated the antistress activity of an ethanolic extract of Withania somnifera root (WS) in mice subjected to stress. Adult male albino mice were treated with the vehicle or WS (23 mg/kg/day, P.O.) for 7 days and subjected to the swim endurance test or cold restraint stress. On day 8, blood was collected from animals subjected to cold restraint stress for analysis. Mice treated with WS showed an increased duration of swimming time in the swim endurance test compared to mice treated with the vehicle. Mice treated with the vehicle and subjected to cold restraint stress showed increased WBC count, blood glucose, plasma cortisol and serum triglycerides compared to mice treated with the vehicle and not subjected to stress. Mice treated with WS and subjected to cold restraint stress showed decreased WBC count, blood glucose, plasma cortisol and serum triglycerides compared to mice treated with the vehicle and subjected to cold restraint stress.

Kaur and coworkers[35] demonstrated the antistress effect of 1-oxo-5β,6β-epoxy-witha-2-ene-27-ethoxy-olide isolated from the roots of Withania somnifera in rats. Male albino Wistar rats treated with this compound (2.5 mg/kg, P.O.) and subjected to cold-hypoxia-restraint (C-H-R) stress showed decreased activities of serum creatine phosphokinase, serum lactate dehydrogenase and serum LPO compared to rats not treated with the compound and subjected to C-H-R stress.

Andrade and coworkers[36] conducted a double-blind, placebo-controlled trial to evaluate the anxiolytic efficacy of an ethanol extract of Withania somnifera (WS). Subjects diagnosed with anxiety disorders were randomly assigned to an experimental group (n=20) and a placebo group (n=19). Subjects in the experimental group received two 250 mg WS tablets twice daily for six weeks. Subjects in the placebo group were treated similarly with placebo tablets. Subjects were tested at baseline, week 2 and week 6. Subjects in the experimental group showed some improvements at week 2 and week 6 compared to baseline. Subjects in the placebo group showed no significant improvement.

Auddy and coworkers[37] evaluated the antistress activity of a standardized Withania somnifera root and leaf extract (WSE) in chronically-stressed humans. In a double-blind, randomized, placebo-controlled study, 130 subjects identified as stressed based on the modified Hamilton Anxiety Scale (mHAM-A) were selected for the study. They were randomly divided into four groups and treated as follows. Each subject was given two bottles of capsules with instructions to take one capsule from bottle 1 before lunch and one capsule from bottle 2 before dinner for 60 days. Bottle 1 given to group 1 contained 125 mg WSE capsules and bottle 2 contained placebo. Both bottles given to groups 2, 3 and 4 contained 125 mg WSE capsules, 250 mg WSE capsules, and placebo respectively. Each subject was tested using the mHAM-A questionnaire at baseline, day 30 and day 60. Blood samples from each subject were collected at baseline and day 60. Placebo group subjects showed no significant change in mHAM-A stress and anxiety scores on days 30 and 60 compared to baseline. All other groups showed a dose-dependent decrease in mHAM-A score on days 30 and 60. On day 60, groups 1, 2 and 3 showed decreased pulse rate, blood pressure, serum cortisol, CRP, TC, TG, LDL-C, HDL-C, and increased DHEAS and hemoglobin compared to the corresponding baseline. The authors concluded that "daily use of WSE would benefit people suffering from the effects of stress and anxiety without any adverse effects".

Chandrashekar and coworkers[38] conducted a double-blind, randomized, placebo-controlled trial to evaluate the efficacy of an extract of Withania somnifera root (WS) in reducing stress and anxiety in adults. 41 men and 23 women (18-54 years old) with a history of chronic stress were selected for the study. The subjects were randomly assigned to an experimental group or placebo group. They were given a blinded kit of capsules and instructed to take one capsule twice a day after meals for 60 days. Capsules given to the experimental group contained 300 mg of WS per capsule, whereas capsules given to the placebo group were a WS lookalike without WS. Subjects were tested on days 0 and 60 using the perceived stress scale (PSS), General Health Questionnaire-28 (GHQ-28) and the Depression Anxiety Stress Scale (DASS). PSS was used to assess self-perception of stress. GHQ-28 assesses somatic stress, anxiety and insomnia, social dysfunction and severe depression. DASS assesses depression, anxiety and stress. Serum cortisol was also measured on days 0 and 60. PSS, GHQ-28 and DASS scores as well as serum cortisol decreased significantly after 60 days in the experimental group, whereas the placebo group did not show significant changes. The authors concluded that "Ashwagandha root extract improves an individual's resistance towards stress and thereby improves self assessed quality of life".

In a double-blind, randomized, placebo-controlled trial, Khyati and Anup[39] evaluated the efficacy of Ashwagandha granules in the management of generalized anxiety disorders (GAD). Subjects in the age group 16-60 years diagnosed with GAD were randomly assigned to treatment and control groups. The subjects were given blinded granules with the instruction to take 4 g granules thrice daily for 60 days. The treatment group received Ashwagandha granules and the controlled group received Ashwagandha lookalike granules. Subjects were tested before and after treatment using the Hamilton Anxiety Rating Scale. No significant changes were observed in the score after the treatment compared to baseline.

Gajarmal and Shende[40] evaluated the antistress effect of Ashwagandha granules in a clinical trial. 40 subjects (35-65 years old) experiencing workplace mental stress were treated with Ashwagandha granules (10 g/day, in two divided doses) for 60 days. The subjects were tested before and after treatment using the workplace stress scale, perceived stress scale, and scales that assessed sleep, anger, sadness and enthusiasm for work. Serum cortisol was also measured on days 0 and 60. After the treatment, the subjects showed considerable improvement.

In a double-blind, randomized, placebo-controlled trial, Choudhary and coworkers[41] evaluated the safety and efficacy of a standardized Ashwagandha root extract in subjects suffering from chronic stress and body weight management issues. Subjects who met the selection criteria (n=52, 38 male and 14 female, 18–60 years of age) were randomly divided into a treatment group (n=26) and control group (n=26). The subjects in the treatment group received 300 mg of a standardized Ashwagandha root extract in capsule form, twice daily with water for 8 weeks. The control group received placebo capsules. At the beginning of the study and at the end of 4 and 8 weeks, the subjects were assessed using the following outcome measures: perceived stress scale (PSS), food cravings questionnaire (FCQ), Oxford happiness questionnaire (OHQ), three-factor eating questionnaire (TEFQ), serum cortisol, body weight and body mass index. At the end of the study, the treatment group showed a significant reduction of mean scores on the PSS, FCQ, OHQ and TEFQ, and a decrease in body weight, body mass index and serum cortisol level. The subjects tolerated the treatment well without serious adverse effects. The authors concluded that "The outcome of this study suggests that Ashwagandha root extract can be used for body weight management in adults under chronic stress".

Lopresti and coworkers[42] conducted a randomized, double-blind, placebo-controlled study to evaluate the effect of Ashwagandha extract (ASH) on stress in healthy adults. 60 adults were randomly placed into an Ashwagandha or placebo group. Subjects in the Ashwagandha group were treated with one 240 mg Ashwagandha capsule per day for 60 days and the placebo group received placebo capsules. After the treatment, the subjects in the Ashwagandha group showed a decrease in HAM-A (Hamilton Anxiety Rating Scale), DASS-21 (Depression, Anxiety, Stress Scale-21) and serum cortisol compared to the placebo group. ASH was well tolerated without adverse effects.

References

1   Depression and other Common Mental Disorders: Global Health Estimates. World Health Organization.
     https://www.who.int/publications-detail/depression-global-health-estimates
2   Facts and Statistics, Anxiety and Depression Association of America.
     https://adaa.org/about-adaa/press-room/facts-statistics
3   Depression, US National Library of Medicine.
     https://medlineplus.gov/depression.html
4   H Selye. Forty years of stress research: principal remaining problems and

misconceptions. CMA Journal (1976) 115: 53-56.

5   J M Koolhaas, A Bartolomucci, B Buwalda, S F de Boer, G Flugge, S M
    Korte, P Meerlo, R Murison, B Olivier, P Palanza, G Richter-Levin, A
    Sgoifo, T Steimer, O Stiedl, G Van Dijk, M Wohr, E Fuchs. Stress revisited:
    A critical evaluation of the stress concept, Neuroscience and Biobehavioral
    Reviews (2011) 35: 1291-1301.

6   S H Scharf, M V Schmidt. Animal models of stress vulnerability and
    resilience in translational research. Curr Psychiatry Rep (2012) 14 (2): 159-
    165.

7   W Beerling, J M Koolhaas, A Ahnaou, J A Bouwknecht, S F de Boer, P
    Meerlo, W H I M Drinkenburg. Physiological and hormonal responses to
    novelty exposure in rats are mainly related to ongoing behavioral activity.
    Physiology and Behavior (2011) 103: 412-420.

8   Sheldon Cohen, Denise Janicki-Deverts, Gregory E Miller. Psychological
    stress and disease. JAMA (2007) 298 (14): 1685-1687.

9   S. K. Bhattacharya, A. Bhattacharya, K. Sairam and S. Ghosal. Anxiolytic-
    antidepressant activity of Withania somnifera glycowithanolides: an
    experimental study. Phytomedicine (2000) 7 (6): 463-469.

10 Giridhari Lal Gupta and Avtar Chand Rana. Effect of Withania somnifera
    Dunal in ethanol-induced anxiolysis and withdrawal anxiety in rats. Indian
    Journal of Experimental Biology (2008) 46: 470-475.

11 Zaved Ahmed Khan and Asit Ranjan Ghosh. Withaferin A displays
    enhanced anxiolytic efficacy without tolerance in rats following sub chronic
    administration. African Journal of Biotechnology (2011) 10 (60): 12973-
    12978.

12 Mohammad Afsal, Sanjiv Karale, Jagadish V Kamath. Evaluation of
    anticonvulsant and antidepressant activity of EPIC-Q TAB: An Ayurvedic
    formulation. Journal of Pharmaceutical and Scientific Innovation (2014) 3 (4):
    397-400.

13 P. C. Shah, N. A. Trivedi, J. D. Bhatt and K. G. Hemavathi. Effect of
    Withania somnifera on forced swimming test induced immobility in mice and
    its interactions with various drugs. Indian J Physiol Pharmacol (2006) 50 (4):
    409-415.

14 T. Maity, A. Adhikari, K. Bhattacharya, S. Biswas, PK Debnath and CS
    Maharana. A study on evaluation of antidepressant effect of imipramine
    adjunct with Ashwagandha and Brahmi. Nepal Med Coll J (2011) 13 (4): 250-
    253.

15 Jayanthi MK, Prathima C, Huralikuppi JC, Suresha RN, and Murali Dhar.
    Anti-depressant effects of Withania somnifera fat (Ashwagandha ghrutha)
    extract in experimental mice. International Journal of Pharma and Bio
    Sciences (2012) 3 (1): 33-42.

16 Yogesh S. Katare, Santosh S. Bhujbal, Anand R. Bafna, Somashekar S.
    Shyale, Maruti K. Shelar, Sagar D. Kadam, Dhananjay A. Landge, and
    Darshan V. Shah, Evaluation of anxiolytic effect of a polyherbal formulation
    in mice. European Journal of Experimental Biology (2012) 2 (6): 2093-2098.

17 Makawana S, Suhagiya B, Bhandari A, Chaudagar K. Antidepressant effects:
    hydroalcoholic extract of Withania somnifera, Berberis aristata and Mucana
    pruriens on tail suspension test in mice. International Journal of
    Pharmaceutical Research and Bio-Science (2014) 3 (4): 815-822.

18 Safora Mirzaei, Sattar Kaikhavani, Gholamreza Mirzaei, Ali Sohrabnezhad,
    Reza Valizadeh. Comparison of anxiolytic effects of root extracts of winter
    cherry (Withania somnifera) with the effects of diazepam in male wistar rats. J
    Bas Res Med Sci (2014) 1 (3): 45-51.

19 P. Bharathi, V. Seshayamma, G. Hari Jagannadharao, N. Sivakumar.

Evaluation of antidepressant activity of aqueous extract of Withania somnifera [Ashwagandha] roots in albino mice. IOSR Journal of Pharmacy and Biological Sciences (2015) 10 (1): 27-29.

20 Gopala Krishna HN, Sangha RB, Misra N, Pai MRSM. Antianxiety activity of NR-ANX-C, a polyherbal preparation in rats. Indian Journal of Pharmacology (2006) 38 (5): 330-335.

21 L. Mohan, U. S, C. Rao, H. N. Gopalakrishna, and V. Nair. Evaluation of the anxiolytic activity of NR-ANX-C (a polyherbal formulation) in ethanol withdrawal-induced anxiety behavior in rats. Evidence Based Complementary and Alternative Medicine, volume 2011, Article ID 327160, 7 pages.

22 Amitabh A Kumar and Reddy Kiran K P. Anxiolytic profile of a polyherbal drug mentat. Int. J. Pharm. Med and Bio. Sc. (2013) 2 (4): 21-27.

23 Kulkarni SK, Verma A. Prevention of development of tolerance and dependence to opiate in mice by BR-A (Mentat), a herbal psychotropic preparation. Indian J Exp Biol (1992) 10: 885-8.

24 Kulkarni SK, Sharma A. Reversal of diazepam withdrawal induced hyperactivity in mice by BR 16-A (Mentat), A herbal formulation. Indian J Exp Biol (1994) 32 (12): 886-8.

25 Shrinivas K Kulkarni, Ipe Ninan. Inhibition of morphine tolerance and dependence by Withania somnifera in mice. Journal of Ethnopharmacology (1997) 57 (3): 213-217.

26 Bhanu PS Kaurav, Manish M Wanjari, Amol Chandekar, Nagendra Singh Chauhan, Neeraj Upamanyu. Influence of Withania somnifera on obsessive compulsive disorder in mice. Asian Pacific Journal of Tropical Medicine (2012) 380-384.

27 N. Singh, R. Nath, A. Lata, S. P. Singh, R. P. Kohli and K. P. Bhargava. Withania somnifera (Ashwagandha), a rejuvenating herbal drug which enhances survival during stress (an adaptogen). Int. J. Crude Drug Res (1982) 20 (1): 29-35.

28 Salil K. Bhattacharya, Raj K. Goel, Ravinder Kaur, Shibnath Ghosal, Anti-stress activity of sitoindosides VII and VIII, new acylsterylglucosides from Withania somnifera. Phytotherapy Research (1987) 1 (1): 32-37.

29 S. K. Bhattacharya, A. V. Muruganandam. Adaptogenic activity of Withania somnifera: an experimental study using a rat model of chronic stress. Pharmacology, Biochemistry and Behavior (2003) 75: 547-555.

30 R. Archana, A. Namasivayam. Antistressor effect of Withania somnifera. Journal of Ethnopharmacology (1999) 64: 91-93.

31 B. Singh, A. K. Saxena, B. K. Chandan, D. K. Gupta, K. K. Bhutani and K. K. Anand. Adaptogenic activity of a novel, withanolide-free aqueous fraction from the roots of Withania somnifera Dun. Phytotherapy Research (2001) 15:311-318.

32 B. Singh, B. K. Chandan and D. K. Gupta. Adaptogenic activity of a novel withanolide-free aqueous fraction from the roots of Withania somnifera Dunn. (part II) Phytotherapy Research (2003) 17: 531-536.

33 H. Jain, S. D. Parial, E. Jarald, Anwar S. Daud, Showkat Ahmad. Extraction of Ashwagandha by conventional methods and evaluation of its antistress activity. International Journal of Green Pharmacy (2010): 183-185.

34 Anju. Adaptogenic and anti-stress activity of Withania somnifera in stress induced mice. Research Journal of Pharmaceutical, Biological and Chemical Sciences (2011) 2 (4): 676-684.

35 Parvinder Kaur, Meenakshi Sharma, Sheenu Mathur, Manisha Tiwari, Harish M. Divekar, Ratan Kumar, Kaushal K. Srivastava and Ramesh Chandra. Effect of 1-oxo-5β, 6β- epoxy-witha-2-ene-27-ethoxy-olide isolated from the roots of Withania somnifera on stress indices in wistar rats. The

Journal of Alternative and Complementary Medicine (2003) 9 (6): 897-907.

36   Chittaranjan Andrade, Anitha Aswath, S. K. Chaturvedi. M. Srinivasa and R. Raguram. A double-blind, placebo-controlled evaluation of the anxiolytic efficacy of an ethanolic extract of Withania somnifera. Indian Journal of Psychiatry (2000) 42(3): 295-301.

37   Biswajit Auddy, Jayaram Hazra, Achintya Mitra, Bruce Abedon, Shibnath Ghosal. A standardized Withania somnifera extract significantly reduces stress-related parameters in chronically stressed humans: a double-blind, randomized, placebo-controlled study. JANA (2008) 11(1): 50-56.

38   K. Chandrasekhar, Jyoti Kapoor, Sridhar Anishetty. A prospective, randomized double-blind, placebo controlled study of safety and efficacy of a high-concentration full-spectrum extract of Ashwagandha root in reducing stress and anxiety in adults. Indian Journal of Psychological Medicine (2012) 34 (3): 255-262.

39   Sud Khyati S and Thaker Anup B. A randomized double blind placebo controlled study of Ashwagandha on generalized anxiety disorder. International Ayurvedic Medical Journal (2013) 1 (5): 1-7.

40   Gajarmal Amit Ashok, Shende M. B. A clinical evaluation of antistress activity of Ashwagandha (Withania somnifera Dunal) on employees experiencing mental stress at work place. International Journal of Ayurveda and Pharma Research (2015) 3 (1): 37-45.

41   Dnyanraj Choudhary, Sauvik Bhattacharya and Kedar Joshi. Body weight management in adults under chronic stress through treatment with Ashwagandha root extract: A double blind, randomized, placebo-controlled trial. Journal of Evidence-Based Complementary & Alternative Medicine (2017) 22 (1): 96-106.

42   Adrian L. Lopresti, Stephen J. Smith, Hakeemudin Malvi, Rahul Kodgule. An investigation into the stress-relieving and pharmacological actions of an ashwagandha (Withania somnifera) extract: A randomized, double-blind, placebo-controlled study. Medicine (Baltimore) 2019; 98 (37): e17186.

6 – Anticonvulsant Activity

6.1 – Introduction

Epilepsy is a chronic brain disorder that is characterized by repeated unprovoked seizures. Seizures are short episodes of uncontrolled behavior caused by abnormal electrical activity in the brain. Seizures can last from a few seconds to several minutes. They vary widely from momentary lapses of attention and muscle jerks to severe and prolonged convulsions[1]. There are several types of seizures, but most can be categorized as either focal or generalized[2]. Focal seizures begin in one small region of the brain, whereas generalized seizures start all over the brain. More than half of all observed epileptic disorders have no identifiable cause. The rest have been attributed to various factors including genetics, head trauma, stroke, heart disease and prenatal injury[1].

More than 50 million people worldwide and about 3.4 million people in the United States have epilepsy[2]. There is currently no cure for epilepsy, but treatments are available to eliminate or reduce seizures. Conventional therapies involve antiepileptic drugs and sometimes surgery. A number of studies have examined the anticonvulsant activity of Withania somnifera and the results are summarized below.

6.2 – Summary of Results

Kulkarni and George[3] reported that chronic treatment of mice with Withania somnifera root extract (WS) provided significant protection against pentylenetetrazole (PTZ)-induced kindling. Laka mice treated with PTZ thrice a week for 9 weeks exhibited CNS excitations and convulsions. Mice treated with WS before the treatment with PTZ showed only a mild degree of CNS excitation and convulsion. The effect of WS (100 mg/kg) was comparable to that of diazepam (1 mg/kg). In a later investigation, Kulkarni and coworkers[4] showed the possible involvement of the GABAergic system for the anticonvulsant effect of WS. Male albino mice treated with WS

(100 or 200 mg/kg, P.O.) and infused with PTZ (iv) showed an increased seizure threshold for the onset of tonic extension compared to controls. Treatment with a lower dose of WS (50 mg/kg, P.O.) showed no such effect. Treatment with WS (50 mg/kg, P.O.) + GABA (25 mg/kg, i.p.) or WS (50 mg/kg, P.O.) + diazepam (0.5 mg/kg, i.p.) increased the seizure threshold compared to controls. The authors concluded that "the anti-convulsant effect of WS in PTZ iv threshold paradigm possibly involved the $GABA_A$ receptor modulation and thus reinforces the use of W. somnifera preparation in reducing the seizure propagation during convulsive episodes".

Kulkarni and coworkers[5] investigated the anticonvulsant action of Withania somnifera root extract (WS) in a lithium-pilocarpine model of status epilepticus (SE). Adult male Wistar rats injected with lithium chloride (3 meq/kg, i.p.) followed by pilocarpine (30 mg/kg S.C.) exhibited SE and 100% mortality. Pretreatment with WS (100 mg/kg, P.O.) delayed the onset of forelimb clonus with rearing but showed no effect on mortality. Pretreatment with diazepam (5 mg/kg, P.O.) or clonazepam (1.0 mg/kg, P.O.) provided full protection. Pretreatment with diazepam (2.5 mg/kg)+ WS (100 mg/kg) or clonazepam (0.5 mg/kg) + WS (100 mg/kg) also provided full protection. Pretreatment with WS (100 mg/kg/day P.O.) for 7 days reduced the mortality to 60%.

Roshanaei and Neda[6] examined the effect of a hydroalcoholic extract of Withania somnifera roots (WSRE) against PTZ-induced seizure threshold in mice. Male mice treated with WSRE (25-100 mg/kg, i.p.) followed by PTZ (i.p.) showed a dose-dependent increase in seizure threshold compared to controls.

Soman and coworkers[7] examined the effects of an aqueous extract of Withania somnifera roots (WS) and withanolide A (WA) on temporal lobe epilepsy (TLE) and associated motor learning impairment in rats. Carbamazepine (CBZ) was also studied for comparison. TLE was induced in male Wistar rats by injecting pilocarpine (350 mg/kg, i.p.). Epileptic rats were treated with saline, WS (100 mg/kg/day, P.O.), WA (10 μmol/kg/day, P.O.) or CBZ (150 mg/kg/day, P.O.) for 15 days. Normal rats treated with saline served as controls. Some rats from each group were subjected to the rotarod, grid walk and narrow beam tests. The remaining rats were sacrificed for biochemical analysis. Epileptic rats treated with the vehicle showed frequent seizures, downregulated retention time (rotarod test), increased footfalls (grid walk test) and decreased retention of balance (narrow beam test) compared to controls. Treatment of epileptic rats with WS or WA reduced the frequency of seizures and reversed the other changes. Treatment of epileptic rats with CBZ significantly reduced the frequency of seizures, upregulated retention time and decreased footfalls, but had no effect on retention of balance. Epileptic rats showed a decreased level of glutamate, downregulation of GAD and GLAST expression, and increased IP3 content in the cerebellum compared to controls. WS- and WA-treated epileptic rats showed a reversal of these changes. CBZ-treated epileptic rats showed a reversal of the changes in glutamate content and GLAST expression. A receptor binding study of [³H] AMPA in the cerebellum of epileptic rats showed decreased AMPA receptor density compared to controls. WS-, WA- and CBZ-treated rats showed a reversal of this change. The authors suggested that "WS and WA regulate AMPA receptor function in the cerebellum of rats with TLE, which has therapeutic application in epilepsy".

Balamurugan and coworkers[8] examined the antiepileptic activity of a polyherbal extract (PHE) containing Withania somnifera as the main ingredient against seizures induced by maximal electroshock (MES) in rats. Adult Wistar albino rats treated with PHE (250 or 500 mg/kg/day, P.O.) for 15 days and subjected to MES showed the following changes compared to rats treated with the vehicle and subjected to MES:

- reduction of various seizure phases and recovery time
- increased levels of serotonin, dopamine and noradrenaline (forebrain)

The effect of PHE was comparable to phenytoin.

Tanna and coworkers[9] studied the protective effect of Ashwagandharishta and Atasi taila alone and in combination against maximal electroshock (MES)-induced seizures in rats. Ashwagandharishta is a polyherbal formulation that contains Withania somnifera as the main ingredient. Atasi taila is the Ayurvedic name for flaxseed oil. Wistar albino rats treated with Atasi taila and subjected to MES showed a decreased flexion phase, fewer convulsions and a shorter recovery time compared to controls (rats treated with distilled water and subjected to MES). Rats treated with Ashwagandharishta showed only a decreased duration of convulsions. Rats treated with Atasi taila + Ashwagandharishta showed a shorter flexion phase and a decreased duration of convulsions.

Afsal and coworkers[10] demonstrated the anticonvulsant activity of Epic-Q in experimental animal models. Epic-Q is a polyherbal formulation that contains Withania somnifera as a major ingredient. Wistar albino rats treated with the formula (500 mg/kg, P.O.) and subjected to MES showed a decreased extension phase compared to rats treated with distilled water and subjected to MES. Albino mice treated with the formula (500 mg/kg/day, P.O.) for 7 days and challenged with isoniazid (300 mg/kg, i.p.) showed a delayed onset of convulsions and tonic phase compared to mice treated with the vehicle and challenged with isoniazid.

Ekambaram[11] investigated the effect of an aqueous extract of Withania somnifera roots (WS) on tolerance to the antiepileptic effect of phenobarbitone (PHB) in mice. Adult Swiss albino mice treated with PHB (25 mg/kg/day, i.p.) for 18 days and subjected to MES on alternate days showed an 80% incidence of tolerance, cognitive impairment and oxidative stress. Mice treated with PHB (25 mg/kg/day, i.p.) + WS (100 mg/kg/day, P.O.) showed a 25% incidence of tolerance and reduced cognitive impairment and oxidative stress.

Salama and coworkers[12] examined the effect of an aqueous extract of Withania somnifera seeds (WS) against pilocarpine-induced convulsions in rats. Adult male Wistar albino rats were given a single dose of pilocarpine (300 mg/kg, i.p.) and used in the study after 15 days. Normal rats served as controls. At the end of the experimental period, the epileptic rats showed the following changes compared to controls:

- decreased antioxidant capacity, decreased activity of Na^+/K^+-ATPase and increased serum Ca levels

- decreased GSH and increased MDA, NO, serotonin and dopamine in the hippocampus

- clusters of injured neurons, vacuolization, shrinking, apoptosis and lysis in the brain

Epileptic rats treated with WS (25 or 50 mg/kg/day) or carbamazepine (100 mg/kg/day) for 15 days showed a reversal of these changes to near control levels. The 50 mg dose of WS was more effective than the 25 mg dose and was comparable to carbamazepine.

Raju and coworkers[13] found that an alcohol extract of Withania somnifera (300 mg/kg, i.p.) was effective against MES- and PTZ-induced epilepsy in albino rats.

References

1   Epilepsy. World Health Organization. https://www.who.int/news-room/fact-sheets/detail/epilepsy

2   Centers for Disease Control and Prevention. Frequently asked questions. https://www.cdc.gov/epilepsy/about/faq.htm

3   S. K. Kulkarni and B. George. Anticonvulsant action of Withania somnifera (Ashwagandha) root extract against pentylenetetrazol-induced kindling in mice. Phytotherapy Research (1996) 10: 447-449.

4   S. K. Kulkarni, Kiran Kumar Akula and Ashish Dhir. Effect of Withania somnifera Dunal root extract against pentylenetetrazol seizure threshold in mice: Possible involvement of GABAergic system. Indian Journal of Experimental Biology (2008) 46: 465-469.

5   S. K. Kulkarni, B. George and R. Mathur. Protective effect of Withania somnifera root extract on electrographic activity in a lithium pilocarpine model of status epilepticus. Phytotherapy Research (1998) 12: 451-453.

6   Kambiz Roshanaei and Nikoklam Nazif Neda. Effect of Withania somnifera root extract on PTZ-induced seizure threshold in mice. Research Journal of Fisheries and Hydrobiology (2015) 10 (10): 719-723.

7   Smijin Soman, T. R. Anju, S. Jayanarayanan, Sherin Antony, C. S. Paulose. Impaired motor learning attributed to altered AMPA receptor function in the cerebellum of rats with temporal lobe epilepsy: Ameliorating effects of Withania somnifera and Withanolide A. Epilepsy & Behavior (2013) 27: 484-491.

8   G. Balamurugan, P. Muralidharan, and S. Selvarajan. Anti epileptic activity of poly herbal extract from Indian medicinal plants. J. Sci. Res (2009) 1 (1): 153-159.

9   Ila R. Tanna, Hetal B. Aghera, B. K. Ashok, H. M. Chandola. Protective role of Ashwagandharishta and flax seed oil against maximal electroshock induced seizures in albino rats. AYU (2012) 33 (1): 114-18.

10 Mohammad Afsal, Sanjiv Karale, Jagadish V Kamath. Evaluation of anticonvulsant and antidepressant activity of EPIC-QTAB: an ayurvedic polyherbal formulation. Journal of Pharmaceutical and Scientific Innovation (2014) 3(4): 397-400.

11 Vijayakumar Andi Ekambaram. Effect of aqueous extract Withania somnifera on tolerance to antiepileptic effect of phenobarbitone in mice. Journal of Young Pharmacists (2015) 7(3): 180-186.

12 Abeer A. A. Salama, Mahitab El-Kassaby, Mohamed E. Elhadidy, Ehab R. Abdel Raouf, Aboelfetoh M. Abdalla, Abdel Razik H. Farrag. Effect of the aqueous seed extract of Withania somnifera (Ashwagandha) against pilocarpine-induced convulsions in rats. Int. J. Pharm. Sci. Rev. Res (2016) 41 (1): 116-121.

13 Santhosh Kumar Raju, Basavanna PL, Nagesh HN, Ajay D Shanbhag. A study on the anticonvulsant activity of Withania somnifera (Dunal) in albino rats. National Journal of Physiology, Pharmacy and Pharmacology (2017) 7 (1): 17-21.

7 – Analgesic Activity

7.1 – Introduction

Pain is an irritating feeling one experiences when exposed to a noxious stimulus (internal or external)[1]. The International Association for the study of Pain (IASP) defines pain as "an unpleasant sensory and emotional experience associated with actual or potential tissue damage or described in terms of such change"[2]. Although pain is uncomfortable, it is a valuable warning signal for potentially health-threatening conditions. The most common drugs used for pain relief are acetaminophen, nonsteroidal anti-inflammatory drugs and opioids. A number of Ayurvedic herbs including Withania somnifera are also used. The results from several investigations reporting the antinociceptive/analgesic effects of Withania somnifera are summarized below.

7.2 – Summary of results

Modi and coworkers[1] studied the analgesic activity of an aqueous extract of Withania somnifera root (WS) in mice and rats. Albino mice and rats were treated with 5 ml/kg saline (control), aspirin, or WS (400, 800, or 1600 mg/kg). The analgesic effect in the mice group was tested by the acetic acid-induced writhing and hot plate tests. In the acetic acid-induced writhing test, mice treated with WS or aspirin (100 mg/kg) showed a decreased writhing response compared to controls. The effect of 1600 mg/kg of WS was similar to 100 mg/kg of aspirin. In the hot plate method, mice treated with WS showed increased reaction times compared to controls. The effect of 1600 mg/kg of WS was similar to 5 mg/kg of the standard tramadol. Rats treated with WS and subjected to the tail flick test showed an increased latency period compared to controls. The effect of 1600 mg/kg of WS was similar to 5 mg/kg of tramadol.

Khalili[3] demonstrated the antinociceptive effect of Withania somnifera WS) in diabetic rats by using the formalin test. Diabetes was induced in male albino Wistar rats by injecting streptozotocin (STZ). Diabetic rats that received rat pellets mixed with WS (6.25 % WS) for two months and subjected to the formalin test showed lower nociceptive scores at both phases of the test compared to controls (diabetic rats not treated with WS). The standard analgesic sodium salicylate (200 mg/kg, i.p.) showed lower nociceptive scores only at the chronic phase of the test. The authors concluded that "these results indicate that two month administration of ashwagandha could attenuate nociceptive score in an experimental model of diabetes mellitus and this may be considered as a potential treatment for painful diabetic neuropathy".

Sabina and coworkers[4] examined the analgesic activity of Withaferin A (WA) by using the acetic acid-induced abdominal constriction and hot plate tests. Swiss albino mice treated with WA (20 or 30 mg/kg, i.p.) or indomethacin (10 mg/kg, i.p) 30 min before injecting 0.6% acetic acid (10 ml/kg, i.p.) showed a reduced number of abdominal constrictions compared to controls (mice treated with saline and injected with acetic acid). Mice treated as before with WA or indomethacin and subjected to the hot plate test showed an increased reaction time compared to controls. WA treatment did not cause gastric damage in mice, whereas indomethacin produced gastric ulcers.

Pradeep and coworkers[5] evaluated the antinociceptive effect of a standardized aqueous extract of Withania somnifera root (WS) in diabetic rats. Male Sprague Dawley rats were injected with STZ (50 mg/kg, i.p.) and waited for 4 weeks for the development of hypersensitivity to pain stimuli. These rats were treated with WS (100 mg/kg/day, P.O.), imipramine (10.5 mg/kg/day, P.O.), fluoxetine (14.5 mg/kg/day, P.O.) or quercetin (10 mg/kg/day, P.O.) for 21 days and subjected to the tail immersion test (cold water), tail immersion test (hot water) or the formalin test. In the tail immersion test (cold water), the WS and drug-treated groups showed increased tail withdrawal latency compared to diabetic controls (diabetic rats not treated with WS or other drugs). In the tail immersion test (hot water), the WS and drug-treated groups showed an increased latency period compared to diabetic controls. In the formalin test, the WS and drug-treated groups showed decreased flinches compared to diabetic controls. The authors concluded that "The results of this pre-clinical study on rats display potential antinociceptive effect of W. somnifera. Data here obtained allows us to propose this plant species as an excellent candidate for isolating new substances with potential antinociceptive effect".

Taznin and coworkers[6] examined the antinociceptive effect of Balarishta, a polyherbal formulation containing Withania somnifera, by using an acetic acid-induced gastric pain model. Swiss albino mice treated with Balarishta (0.3, 1.0 or 1.5 ml/kg, P.O.) showed a reduction in the number of abdominal constrictions compared to controls. The percent reductions of constrictions were 41.4, 44.8 and

55.2 at 0.3, 1.0 and 55.2 mg/kg respectively. The standard drug aspirin (200 mg/kg) showed a 37.9% reduction. Balarishta at the dose of 0.1 mg/kg did not show a significant reduction in the number of abdominal constrictions, whereas Balarishta (0.1 mg/kg) + aspirin (200 mg/kg) caused a 58.6% reduction.

Shahriar and coworkers[7] investigated the analgesic activity of methanol, ethanol and chloroform extracts of Withania somnifera root in mice by using the acetic acid writhing and tail immersion tests. Swiss albino mice were treated with 1% tween 80 (10 ml/kg, i.p), diclofenac sodium (100 mg/kg, P.O.), methanol extract (100 or 150 mg/kg, P.O.), ethanol extract (100 or 150 mg/kg, P.O.) or chloroform extract (100 or 150 mg/kg, p.o.). Thirty minutes later 0.7% acetic acid (10 ml/kg, i.p.) was injected. Diclofenac sodium and all extracts inhibited writhing compared to controls. The percent reductions in inhibition were 16.61, 70.56, 38.13 and 25.55 for methanol (150 mg/kg), ethanol (150 mg/kg), chloroform (150 mg/kg) and diclofenac sodium (100 mg/kg) respectively. In the tail immersion test, diclofenac sodium and the extracts showed an increased basal reaction time compared to controls. The effect decreased in the following order: diclofenac sodium > ethanol > chloroform > methanol.

Dey and coworkers[8] examined the analgesic activity of a standardized extract of Withania somnifera root (WSR) in stressed mice. WSR was prepared by combining methanol and water extracts of Withania somnifera root in proper proportion to obtain an extract with 2.7% (w/w) withanolides. Male Wistar rats were treated with 0.3% CMC (10 ml/kg/day, P.O.) or WSR (10, 20 or 40 mg/kg/day, P.O.) for 11 days. On the 1st, 5th, 7th and 10th day of treatment, the rats were given a foot shock followed by a hot plate test. Only the WSR- (40 mg/kg) treated group exhibited an analgesic effect on the first day of treatment compared to controls. The efficacy increased dose-dependently with the number of days treated. On the last day, the WSR-treated groups (including the 10 mg/kg group) showed an increased reaction time compared to controls.

Nalini and coworkers[2] conducted a randomized, double-blind, placebo-controlled crossover study to evaluate the analgesic efficacy of a standardized aqueous extract of Withania somnifera (WS). A hot air analgesiometer was used to induce thermal pain on the volar surface of subjects' forearms. Twelve subjects were randomized into two groups: WS and placebo. The pain threshold time of the subjects was determined using the hot air analgesiometer. The subjects in the WS group were given two capsules of WS (500 mg WS/capsule) with water and the placebo group received placebo capsules. Three hours later, the pain threshold time was determined. The procedure was repeated with reversed treatment after two weeks of washout. The WS group showed an increased pain threshold time compared to baseline and the placebo group. The subjects tolerated the treatment without adverse side effects.

Krishna Murthy[9] and coworkers evaluated the analgesic activity of a standardized aqueous extract of Withania somnifera (WS) in healthy human subjects using a mechanical pain model. Twelve healthy male subjects were randomized into two groups: WS and placebo. The subjects in the WS group were treated with two WS capsules (500 mg WS/capsule) and the placebo group received placebo capsules. Mechanical pain was assessed by the Randall-Selitto test before and three hours after the treatment. The process was repeated by reversing the treatment between the groups after 15 days of washout. The WS group showed increased pain threshold force and time as well as increased pain tolerance force and time compared to the placebo group.

Ramakanth and coworkers[10] conducted a randomized, double-blind, placebo-controlled study to evaluate the efficacy and tolerability of a standardized aqueous extract of Withania somnifera (WS) in patients with knee pain. Sixty subjects with knee joint pain were randomized into three groups: 1) WS 250 mg; 2) WS 125 mg; 3) Placebo. The subjects in the first group took 2 capsules (250 mg WS/capsule) a day (one after each meal with water) for 12 weeks. Subjects in the second and third groups consumed 125 mg WS capsules and placebo, respectively, in the same way as the first group. Paracetamol (650 mg) tablets were used as and when required. Assessment was done by the modified Western Ontario and McMaster University Osteoarthritis Index (mWOMAC), Knee Swelling Index (KSI), and Visual Analogue Scale (VAS). At the end of 12 weeks, the first and second groups showed reduced mWOMAC scores, KSI scores and VAS scores for pain, stiffness and disability compared to baseline and the placebo group. The reduction of scores in the first group was greater than the second. The average number of paracetamol tablets used was 10, 13 and 17 in the first, second and third group respectively. The treatment was well tolerated without adverse side effects.

References

1   Pankaj Kumar Modi, Vipin Kumar, Neetu Jain, Saurabh Kohli, Uma Advani. Evaluation of analgesic activity of Withania somnifera in albino rats: an experimental study. International Research Journal of Pharmaceuticals and Applied Sciences (2012) 2 (6): 226-229.

2   P. Nalini, K. Manjunath. N, K. SunilKumar Reddy, P. Usharani. Evaluation of the analgesic activity of standardized aqueous extract of Withania somnifera in healthy human volunteers using Hot air Pain Model. Research Journal of Life Sciences (2013) 1 (2): 1-6.

3   Mohsen Khalili. The effect of oral administration of Withania somnifera root on formalin-induced pain in diabetic rats. Basic and Clinical Neuroscience (2009) 1 (1): 29-31.

4   Evan Prince Sabina, Sonal Chandel, Mahaboob Khan Rasool. Evaluation of analgesic, antipyretic and ulcerogenic effect of Withaferin A. International Journal of Integrative Biology (2009) 6 (2): 52-56.

5   Pradeep S, Prem Kumar N, Deepak Kumar Khajuria, Srinivas Rao G. Preclinical evaluation of antinociceptive effect of Withania somnifera (Ashwagandha) in diabetic peripheral neuropathic rat model. Pharmacologyonline (2010) 2: 283-298.

6   Inin Taznin, Md. Tanvir Morshed, M. Maruf Hassan, Shirin Akhter, Ishtiaq Ahmed, Sanjida Haque, A. B. M. Anwarul Bashar, Mohammed Rahmatullah. Assessment of antinociceptive potentials of two Ayurvedic herbal preparation Balarishta and Sarivadyarishta. Advances in Natural and Applied Sciences (2013) 7 (5): 526-531.

7   Mohammad Shahriar, Fariha Alam and Mir Muhammad Nasir Uddin. Analgesic and neuropharmacological activity of Withania somnifera root. International Journal of Pharmacy (2014) 4 (2): 203-208.

8   Amitabha Dey, Shyam Sunder Chatterjee, Vikas Kumar. Analgesic activity of a Withania somnifera extract in stressed mice. Oriental Pharmacy and Experimental Medicine (2016) 16 (4): 295-302.

9   Manjunath Nookala Krishna Murthy, Srinivas Gundagani, Chandrashekhar Nutalapati, Usharani Pingali. Evaluation of analgesic activity of standardised aqueous extract of Withania somnifera in healthy human volunteers using mechanical pain model. Journal of Clinical and Diagnostic Research (2019) 13 (1): 1-4.

10 G. S. H. Ramakanth, C. Uday Kumar, P. V. Kishan, P. Usharani. A randomized double blind placebo controlled study of efficacy and tolerability of Withania somnifera extracts in knee joint pain. Journal of Ayurveda and Integrative Medicine (2016) 7: 151-157.

8 – Effects on Alcohol and Opioid Tolerance and Addiction

8.1 – Introduction

Tolerance to alcohol and opioids occurs with repeated use over time. This means that a higher quantity of the substance is needed to obtain the same effect achieved initially with a lower quantity[1]. If a person experiences withdrawal symptoms as a result of stopping the use of alcohol/drugs, she/he is said to have developed dependence[1]. The withdrawal symptoms can be mild or excruciating. Often, prolonged use of alcohol or opioids leads to addiction. People with addiction cannot stop the use of alcohol or drugs even after knowing that such actions have terrible consequences[2]. Addiction to alcohol/opioids is a serious global issue. In the US, over 20 million people suffer from alcohol and drug addiction[3]. A variety of treatment options are available for treating addiction. A number of investigations have examined the effect of Withania somnifera on alcohol and opioid tolerance and addiction. The results from some studies are summarized below.

8.2 – Summary of Results

Kulkarni and Verma[4] reported that treatment of mice with BR-16A (20-500 mg/kg/day) prior to the administration of morphine (10 mg/kg/day) for 9 days reduced the development of tolerance to the analgesic effect of morphine (10 mg/kg) in a dose-dependent manner. BR-16A is a polyherbal formulation containing Withania somnifera root. In another study, Kulkarni and Verma[5] examined the effect of BR-16A on alcohol abstinence-induced anxiety and convulsions. Rats and mice receiving ethanol (2-5 g/kg, P.O.) for 6 days showed withdrawal anxiety after stopping ethanol. Treatment with BR-A (100 mg/kg) prior to ethanol administration for 6 days prevented alcohol withdrawal anxiety. Administration of pentylenetetrazole (PTZ, 40 or 60 mg/kg) at a dose below the convulsive threshold to ethanol-withdrawn rats and mice caused convulsions and mortality, whereas BR-16A treatment of alcohol-withdrawn rats and mice prevented reduction of the PTZ threshold. The authors concluded that "the results suggest the usefulness of this safe herbal psychotropic preparation in the management of ethanol withdrawal reactions".

Kulkarni and Sharma[6] investigated the effect of BR-16A on diazepam withdrawal-induced hyperactivity in mice. Mice treated with diazepam (20 mg/kg/day) for 21 days showed hyperactivity on abrupt termination of diazepam. Mice treated with BR-16A (100 and 500 mg/kg/day) and diazepam (20 mg/kg/day) for 21 days showed a reduction of withdrawal-induced hyperactivity. The authors concluded that "BR-16A with its CNS profile of activity could be useful preparation in the management of substance abuse".

Kulkarni and Ninan[7] reported that an extract of Withania somnifera root (WS) inhibited the development of morphine tolerance and dependence in mice. Albino mice that received morphine (10 mg/kg) twice daily for 9 days exhibited maximum analgesia on days 1 and 3, and tolerance on days 9 and 10 of testing. Mice treated with WS (100 mg/kg) and morphine (10 mg/kg) for 9 days as before showed maximum analgesia on all testing days, indicating that WS pretreatment prevented the development of morphine tolerance. Mice treated with morphine for 9 days exhibited escape jumps after naloxone (2 mg/kg) administration on day 10, an indication of dependence development. Mice treated with WS and morphine did not show escape jumps. The authors concluded that "WS is a safe non analgesic herbal preparation which can be used in the treatment of opiate addiction".

Ramarao and coworkers[8] reported that sitoindosides VII-X in combination with Withaferin A from Withania somnifera reversed morphine-induced inhibition of intestinal motility and tolerance to analgesia in mice.

Gupta and Rana[9] examined the effect of an ethanol extract of Withania somnifera root (WS) on ethanol withdrawal anxiety in rats. Male Wistar albino rats that were given alcohol in a liquid diet (9% v/v) for 15 days and stopped receiving alcohol showed alcohol withdrawal anxiety. Administration of WS (100 to 500 mg/kg, P.O.) attenuated withdrawal anxiety in a dose-dependent manner.

Mohan and coworkers[10] evaluated the anxiolytic activity of NR-ANX-C, a polyherbal formulation containing Withania somnifera extract (WS), on ethanol withdrawal-induced anxiety in rats. Male Wistar albino rats were given ethanol (7.5% v/v) instead of drinking water for 10 days and alcohol was substituted by drinking water for 72 hours. These rats exhibited alcohol withdrawal anxiety (elevated plus maze and bright and dark arena tests). Rats treated with WS (40 mg/kg) along with alcohol for 10 days showed a significant reduction in alcohol withdrawal-induced anxiety. The effect of WS (40 mg/kg) was comparable to alprazolam (0.08 mg/kg). The authors concluded that "the polyherbal formulation NR-ANX-C has the potential to be used as an alternative to benzodiazepines in the treatment of ethanol withdrawal".

Ruby and coworkers[11] examined the effect of Withania somnifera root extract (ASW) on alcohol withdrawal syndrome in rats. Albino mice of either sex were given ethanol (2 g/kg/day, oral intubation) for one week and alcohol was withdrawn. These mice exhibited convulsions with a subconvulsive dose of pentylenetetrazole (PTZ), increased immobility time in the fast swim test, and a decreased number of lines crossed in the open field test compared to controls (mice treated with water). Treatment of mice with ethanol+ASW (500 mg/kg/day) or diazepam (1 mg/kg/day) suppressed the PTZ kindling seizures, decreased immobility time in the fast swim test, and increased the number of lines crossed in the open field test compared to alcohol-only treated mice. The authors concluded that "ASW can be used as a safe drug in alcohol withdrawal conditions as a reliable alternative to commonly used BZD class of drugs".

Peana and coworkers[12] found that treatment of adult male Wistar rats with Withania somnifera root extract (WSE) reduced the motivation for drinking and seeking alcohol. The authors suggested that "the use of WSE could represent an interesting and alternative phytotherapic approach for the treatment of excessive alcohol drinking and to prevent alcohol relapse in human alcoholics".

Orru and coworkers[13] reported that pretreatment of male CD1 mice with a standardized extract of Withania somnifera root (WSE, 100 mg/kg, i.p.) prolonged morphine-induced (5 or 10 mg/kg) analgesia and prevented the development of hyperalgesia. WSE also exhibited a high affinity for $GABA_A$ and moderate affinity for $GABA_B$, NMDA and δ opioid receptors. The authors concluded that "This study suggests the therapeutic potential of WSE as a valuable adjuvant agent in opioid-sparing therapies".

Bansal and Banerjee[14] reported that acute administration of Ashwagandha, Shilajit, or a combination of the two prevented alcohol withdrawal anxiety in mice. Chronic administration decreased ethanol intake and increased water intake. Chronic administration of Ashwagandha increased corticohippocampal serotonin levels and GABA levels in the brain. Chronic administration of Shilajit increased corticohippocampal dopamine levels. The authors concluded that "Ashwagandha and Shilajit mediated dose-dependent decrease in ethanol withdrawal anxiety as well as a reduction in ethanol intake in mice. The primary mechanism responsible for anti-addictive activity of Ashwagandha was found via GABAergic and serotonergic system while Shilajit primarily mediated its effect by modulating dopamine levels in mice".

Kotagale and coworkers[15] observed that Withaferin A reduced the signs of alcohol abstinence in rats. Adult Sprague Dawley rats were given alcohol for 21 days. After stopping alcohol, they showed increased somatic behaviors, anxiety and depression. Rats treated with ethanol for 14 days followed by treatment with ethanol and Withaferin A (10-20 mg/kg/day, i.p.) from day 15 to 21 showed a reversal of alcohol withdrawal symptoms. Withaferin A also reduced the elevated plasma corticosterone and ACTH observed in ethanol-withdrawn rats. The authors concluded that "The data clearly projects Withaferin A as a new potential therapeutic intervention in alcohol abuse associated complications".

References

1   The Neurobiology of Drug Addiction. National Institute on Drug Abuse (2007). https://www.drugabuse.gov/sites/default/files/1922-the-neurobiology-of-drug-addiction.pdf

2   Addiction and Substance Use Disorders. American Psychiatric Association (2017). https://www.psychiatry.org/patients-families/addiction

3   Statistics on Addiction in America. Addiction Center. https://www.addictioncenter.com/addiction/addiction-statistics/

4   S. K. Kulkarni and A. Verma. Prevention of tolerance and dependence to opiate in mice by BR-A (Mentat), a herbal psychotropic preparation. Indian J Exp Biol (1992) 30 (10): 885-888.

5   S. K. Kulkarni and A. Verma. Protective effect of BR-16A (Mentat), a herbal preparation on alcohol abstinence-induced anxiety and convulsions. Indian J Exp Biol (1993) 31 (5): 435-439.

6   S. K. Kulkarni and A. Sharma. Reversal of diazepam withdrawal induced hyperactivity in mice by BR-A (mentat), a herbal preparation. Indian J Exp Biol (1994) 32 (12): 886-888.

7   S. K. Kulkarni and I. Ninan. Inhibition of morphine tolerance and dependence by Withania somnifera in mice. Journal of Ethnopharmacology (1997) 57 (3): 213-217.

8   P. Ramarao, K. T.Rao, R. S. Srivastava, S. Ghosal. Effects of glycowithanolides from Withania somnifera on morphine-induced inhibition of intestinal motility and tolerance to analgesia in mice. Phytotherapy Research (1995) 9 (1): 66-68.

9   Girdhari Lal Gupta and Avtar Chand Rana. Effect of Withania somnifera Dunal in ethanol-induced anxiolysis and withdrawal anxiety in rats, Indian Journal of Experimental Biology (2008) 46: 470-475.

10   L. Mohan, U. S. C, Rao, H. N. Gopalkrishna and V. Nair. Evaluation of the anxiolytic activity of NR-ANX-C (a polyherbal formulation) in ethanol withdrawal-induced behavior in rats. Evidence-Based complementary and Alternate medicine, volume 2011, Article ID 327160, 7 pages.

11   Ruby B, Benson MK, Kumar EP, Sudha S, Wilking JE. Evaluation of Ashwagandha in alcohol withdrawal syndrome. Asian Pacific Journal of Tropical Disease (2012) S856-860.

12   Alessandra T. Peana, Giulia Muggironi, Liliana Spina, Michela Rosas, Sanjay B. Kasture, Elisabetta Cotti and Elio Acquas. Effects of Withania somnifera on oral ethanol self-administration in rats. Behavioral Pharmacology (2014) 25 (7): 618-628.

13   Alessandro Orru, Giorgio Marchese, Gianluca Casu, Maria Antonietta Casu, Sanjay Kasture, Filippo Cottiglia, Elio Acquas, Maria Paola Mascia, Nicola Anzani, Stefania Ruiu. Withania somnifera root extract prolongs analgesia and suppresses hyperalgesia in mice treated with morphine. Phytomedicine (2014) 21: 745-752.

14   Priya Bansal and Sugato Banerjee. Effect of Withania Somnifera and Shilajit on Alcohol Addiction in Mice. Pharmacognosy Magazine (2016) 12 (46): 121-128.

15   Nandkishor Ramdas Kotagale, Ankit Kedia, Rupali Gite, Shubham Nilkanth Rahmatkar, Dinesh Yugraj Gawande, Milind Janraoji Umekar, Brijesh Gulabrao Taksande. Withaferin A attenuates alcohol abstinence signs in rats. Pharmacognosy Journal (2018) 10 (6): 1190-1195.

9 – Effect on Insomnia

9.1 – Introduction

Insomnia is a major sleep disorder. People with insomnia have difficulty falling asleep, staying asleep, or both. The prevalence of insomnia ranges from 12% to 20% in the general population and 30% to 48% in the elderly[1]. Nonpharmacological treatments include relaxation techniques, improving sleep hygiene and cognitive behavior therapy. Pharmacological treatments include benzodiazepine sedatives, nonbenzodiazepine sedatives, melatonin receptor agonists, antidepressants, and orexin receptor antagonists.[2]. Many herbal remedies for insomnia are also available. Withania somnifera is commonly used in ayurveda and other practices to treat insomnia; the Latin term "somnifera" means sleep-inducing. A number of scientific investigations have been conducted to evaluate the efficacy of Withania somnifera for insomnia and results from some studies are presented below.

9.2 – Summary of Results

Kumar and Kalonia[3] studied the effect of a Withania somnifera root extract (WS) in sleep-disturbed mice. The grid suspended over water method was used to cause sleep deprivation. Mice deprived of sleep for 48 hours showed decreased body weight, increased anxiety, impaired locomotor activity and oxidative stress (increased LPO and nitrite and decreased glutathione and catalase in brain homogenate) compared to controls (mice not subjected to sleep deprivation). Mice treated with WS (100 or 200 mg/kg/day, P.O.) or diazepam (0.5 mg/kg/day, i.p.) for 5 days and subjected to sleep deprivation on days 4 and 5 showed a reversal of these changes. Administering 100 mg of WS+0.5 mg of diazepam was more effective than 100 mg WS or 0.5 mg diazepam alone. The authors suggested that "Withania somnifera root extract can be used in the management of sleep loss and their related behavioral and biochemical alterations". A subsequent study[4] investigated the effect of Withania somnifera on the sleep-wake cycle of sleep-disturbed rats. Electrodes were implanted in male Wistar rats for polygraphic electroencephalogram (EEG) and electromyogram (EMG) recording.

The rats were allowed one week to recover before being used in the study. Rats deprived of sleep for 24 hours showed delayed sleep latency, reduced slow-wave, REM, and total sleep times, and increased total waking time compared to rats that received normal sleep. Rats treated with WS (100 mg/kg, i.p.) or diazepam (0.5 mg/kg, i.p.) and deprived of sleep for 24 hours showed a reversal of the changes induced by sleep deprivation. Treatment with 100 mg WS+0.5 mg diazepam did not make further improvements compared to 100 mg of WS or 0.5 mg of diazepam. By studying the effect of GABAergic modulators (flumazenil, picrotoxin and muscimol) alone and in combination with WS on electrophysiological parameters, the authors showed the involvement of a GABAergic mechanism in the sleep-promoting effect of WS in a sleep-deprived state.

Manchanda and coworkers[5] examined the effect of an aqueous extract of Withania somnifera leaves (ASH-WEX) on anxiety, cognitive deficits and motor dysfunction in sleep-deprived rats. Wistar albino female rats were divided into three groups: 1) vehicle-treated undisturbed sleep (VUD); 2) vehicle-treated sleep-deprived (VSD); 3) ASH-WEX-treated sleep-deprived (WSD). Groups 1 and 2 were treated with water and group 3 was treated with ASH-WEX (140 mg/kg/day, P.O.) for 15 days. On day 15, groups 2 and 3 were deprived of sleep for 12 hours. The animals were then subjected to the novel object recognition (NORT) and rotarod tests. The VSD group spent less time exploring objects with significantly fewer episodes with new objects and spent more time grooming themselves compared to the VUD group, indicating anxiety-like behavior and impairment of recognition memory due to sleep deprivation. The WSD group spent more time exploring the objects with more episodes with new objects and spent less time grooming themselves compared to the VSD group, indicating a suppression of anxiety-like behavior and improved memory and cognitive functions in sleep-deprived rats. The authors concluded that "The data suggests that Ashwagandha may be a potential agent to suppress the acute effects of sleep loss on learning and memory impairments and may emerge as a novel supplement to control SD-induced cognitive impairments". In a subsequent investigation, Kaur and coworkers[6] examined the effect of ASH-WEX on anxiety and immunomodulation in acute sleep-deprived rats. Wistar albino rats were divided into the VUD, VSD and WSD groups as before and treated in the same way. After 12 hours of sleep deprivation, the animals were subjected to the elevated plus maze test and then used for testing inflammatory and apoptotic markers in the piriform cortex and hippocampus. In the elevated plus maze test, the VSD group showed higher anxiety levels than the VUD group. The WSD group showed behavior similar to the VUD group. ASH-WEX pretreatment of sleep-deprived rats modulated the sleep deprivation-induced expression of inflammatory and immune response markers as well as sleep deprivation-induced apoptosis. The authors concluded that "The current study provides a scientific validation to the anxiolytic, anti-inflammatory and anti-apoptotic properties of Withania somnifera and this medicinal plant may be recommended as a suitable dietary supplement to ameliorate the negative effects associated with sleep deprivation".

Kaushik and coworkers[7] evaluated the effect of alcoholic and water extracts of Ashwagandha leaves on sleep regulation by recording EEG and EMG data in mice. Male C57BL/6 mice treated with the ethanol extract (200 mg/kg, P.O.) showed no change in NREM or REM sleep compared with vehicle (5% DMSO, P.O.)-treated mice, suggesting that Withanolides (major components of the alcohol extract) might not be involved in sleep promotion. Treatment with the water extract increased NREM sleep significantly, with a slight change in REM sleep compared to vehicle-treated mice. Also, administering triethylene glycol (TEG, 10-30 mg) increased NREM sleep in a dose-dependent manner compared to the vehicle-treated group. TEG is a component of the water extract. The authors concluded that "Here we showed that a sleep-promoting active component present in Ashwagandha leaves is TEG and validated the sleep inducing potential of TEG by animal experiments. Further studies are needed to delineate its molecular targets and sleep-promoting pathways".

Langade and coworkers[8] conducted a randomized, double-blind, placebo-controlled study to evaluate the efficacy and safety of a Withania somnifera root extract for insomnia and anxiety. 60 patients with insomnia were randomized into a test group (n=40) and placebo group (n=20). The subjects in the test group were treated with two capsules of the extract (300 mg/capsule) daily with water or milk for 10 weeks. The subjects in the placebo group were treated similarly with lookalike capsules containing starch. All subjects were evaluated at the screening, baseline, 5th and 10th week using sleep actigraphy, the Pittsburgh Sleep Quality Index (PSQI) and the Hamilton anxiety rating scale (HAM-A). The subjects were also asked to maintain a sleep log. The test group showed overall sleep improvement and reduction of anxiety compared to its baseline and the placebo group. The subjects tolerated the treatment without adverse side effects.

References

1   Dhaval Patel, Joel Steinberg, Pragnesh Patel. Insomnia in the elderly: a
    review. Journal of Clinical Sleep Medicine (2018) 14 (6): 1017-1024.
2   Kate Romero, Balaji Goparaju, Kathryn Russo, M Brandon Westover, Matt
    T Bianchi. Alternative remedies for insomnia: a proposed method for
    personalized therapeutic trials. Nature and Science of Sleep (2017) 9: 97-108.
3   Anil Kumar & Harikesh Kalonia. Protective effect of Withania somnifera
    Dunal on the behavioral and biochemical alterations in sleep-disturbed mice
    (Grid over water suspended method). Indian Journal of Experimental
    Biology (2007) 45: 524-528.
4   A. Kumar and H. Kalonia. Effect of Withania somnifera on sleep-wake cycle
    in sleep- disturbed rats: possible GABAergic mechanism. Indian J Pharm Sci
    (2008) 70 (6): 806-810.
5   Shaffi Manchanda, Rachana Mishra, Rumani Singh, Taranjeet Kaur,
    Gurucharan Kaur. Aqueous leaf extract of Withania somnifera as a potential
    neuroprotective agent in sleep-deprived rats: a mechanistic study. Mol
    Neurobiol (2017) 54 (4): 3050-3061.
6   Taranjeet Kaur, Harpal Singh, Rachana Mishra, Shaffi Manchanda, Muskan
    Gupta, Vedangana Saini, Anuradha Sharma, Gurucharan Kaur. Withania
    somnifera as a potential anxiolytic and immunomodulatory agent in acute
    sleep deprived female Wistar rats. Mol Cell Biochem (2017) 427 (1-2): 91-
    101.
7   Mahesh K. Kaushik, Sunil C. Kaul, Renu Wadhwa, Masashi Yanagisawa,
    Yoshihiro Urade. Triethylene glycol, an active component of Ashwagandha
    (Withania somnifera) leaves, is responsible for sleep induction. PLOS ONE
    (2017) 12 (2): e0172508.
8   Deepak Langade, Subodh Kanchi, Jaising Salve, Khokan Debnath, Dhruv
    Ambegaokar. Efficacy and safety of Ashwagandha (Withania somnifera) root
    extract in insomnia and anxiety: a randomized, placebo-controlled study.
    Cureus 11(9): e5797. doi:10.7759/cureus.5797

10 – Anticancer Activity

10.1 – Introduction

Cancer is undoubtedly a life-threatening disease. It is the second leading cause of death across the globe. An estimated 18.1 million new cases of cancer and 9.6 million deaths due to cancer were expected to occur in 2018[1]. The global cancer burden is expected to rise due to several factors including the increasing aging population, lifestyle changes and environmental factors[2]. The good news is that there have been significant advances in research to prevent and treat cancer.

Cancer is not just one disease. It is a group of diseases characterized by the uncontrolled growth and spread of abnormal cells. Normal cells follow an orderly path of growth, division and death, but this process gets disturbed sometimes (e.g. by mutations in the DNA of a cell). When this happens, cells do not die when they should (apoptosis) and new cells do not form as they should. These abnormal cells may form a mass of tissue called a tumor, which can be benign (noncancerous) or malignant (cancerous). Benign tumors tend to grow slowly and do not spread. Whereas cells in malignant tumors invade and destroy nearby normal tissues, and subsequently spread throughout the body (metastasis). Cancers are classified by the location in the body or type of tissue initially affected. Medical professionals frequently refer to cancer by its histological type: carcinoma, sarcoma, myeloma, leukemia, lymphoma, etc[3]. Cancers are typically labeled by stages from I to IV, with IV being the most serious.

The main treatments for cancer are surgery, chemotherapy and radiation therapy. Other treatments include hormonal therapy, targeted therapy and stem cell transplants. Treatment selection depends on the type and stage of cancer, patient age, health status and other personal characteristics. Most people receive a combination of treatments.

The scientific literature reveals the anticancer activity of Withania somnifera against several types of cancer. This is summarized in the following sections.

10.2 – Breast Cancer

Breast cancer is the most commonly occurring cancer in women worldwide. An estimated two million new cases of breast cancer were expected to be diagnosed in 2018[4]. The outlook for women with breast cancer is improving. Survival rates from breast cancer have increased since 1990 due to greater awareness, opportunities for early detection, and availability of effective treatments. However, this does not mean the battle against breast cancer is over. There is still much work to be done.

Traditionally, most breast cancers have been classified as ductal or lobular. Lobular carcinomas start in the lobules, the milk-producing glands. Ductal carcinomas start in the ducts that carry milk from the lobules to the nipples[5]. Breast cancer that is negative for the expression of estrogen (ER), progesterone (PR) and human epidermal growth factor receptor 2 (HER-2) is called triple-negative breast cancer (TNBC)[6]. TNBC is more aggressive than other forms.

Treatments for breast cancer include surgery, radiation therapy, chemotherapy, hormone therapy and targeted therapy. A number of investigations have shown the therapeutic potential of Withania somnifera in breast cancer. Results from some studies are summarized below.

Jayaprakasam and coworkers[7] isolated several compounds listed below from Withania somnifera leaves (Table 10.1) and tested their antiproliferative activity in the human breast cancer cell line MCF-7.

1	Withaferin A
2	Sitoindoside IX
3	4-(1-hydroxy-2,2-dimethylcyclopropanone)-2,3-dihydrowithaferin A
4	2,3-dihydrowithaferin A
5	24,25-dihydro-27-desoxywithaferin A
6	Physagulin D (1→6)-β-D-glucopyranosyl(1→4)-β-D-glucopyranoside
7	27-O-β-D-glucopyranosylphysagulin D
8	Physagulin D
9	Withanoside IV
10	27-O-β-D-glucopyranosylviscosalactone B
11	4,16-dihyroxy-5β,6β-epoxyphysagulin D
12	Viscosalactone B

Table 10.1: Compounds isolated from Withania somnifera leaves

These compounds and diacetylwithaferin A were tested for their antiproliferative activity in breast cancer cells (MCF-7). Except for compounds 7 and 8, they all showed significant growth inhibitory activity. IC_{50} values ranged from 0.27 µg/ml (Withaferin A) to 18.20 µg/ml (compound 6). IC_{50} for the standard adriamycin was 0.36 µg/ml. The authors suggested that "Withania somnifera leaves may be a potential source for the development of cancer therapeutics".

Subbaraju and coworkers[8] isolated a dimeric withanolide, ashwagandhanolide, from the roots of Withania somnifera. This compound was found to inhibit the growth of MCF-7 human breast cancer cells (IC_{50} = 1.45 µg/ml). The authors suggested that "the consumption of Withania somnifera root extract may be beneficial in preventing the progression of certain tumors".

Mulabagal and coworkers[9] isolated Withanolide sulfoxide from Withania somnifera roots and demonstrated its ability to inhibit the proliferation of breast cancer cells (MCF-7). In a dose-response study (0.45-7.5 µg/ml), IC_{50} was found to be 1.26 µg/ml.

Neema and coworkers[10] found that a hydro-alcoholic (1:1) extract of Withania somnifera leaves was cytotoxic to MCF-7 cells. Treatment of MCF-7 cells with the extract inhibited growth in a concentration-dependent manner (IC_{50} = 0.1 µg/ml).

Kaileh and coworkers[11] found that a dichloromethane-methanol (1:1 V/V) extract of Withania somnifera was cytotoxic to MCF-7 (IC_{50} = 60 µg/ml) and MDA-MB-231 (IC_{50} = 200 µg/ml) breast cancer cells.

Stan and coworkers[12] found that treatment of human breast cancer cell lines MCF-7 (estrogen positive) and MDA-MB-231 (estrogen independent) with Withaferin A (0.5-3 µg/ml) decreased cell survival in a dose-dependent manner by inducing apoptosis. Withaferin A-induced apoptosis was accompanied by the induction of Bim-s, a short form of the Bim protein that induces apoptosis. The induction of Bim-S was FOXO3a-dependent. An in vivo study showed that pretreatment with Withaferin A inhibited the growth of MDA-MB-231 xenografts in female athymic mice by inducing apoptosis. Another publication[13] reported that Withaferin A treatment of MDA-MB-231 and MCF-7 cell lines caused irreversible cell cycle arrest in the G2-M phase.

Lee and coworkers[14] demonstrated that Withaferin A inhibited activation of Signal Transducer and Activator of Transcription 3 (STAT3) in human breast cancer cells. STAT3 has been implicated in the initiation and progression of many types of cancer, including breast cancer. Treatment of MDA-MB-231 cells with Withaferin A inhibited phosphorylation of STAT3 (Tyr^{705}) and decreased its protein level, inhibited the phosphorylation of JAK2 and its protein level, as well as decreased STAT3-STAT3 dimerization and nuclear translocation. In both the MDA-MB-231 and MCF-7 cells, Withaferin A treatment inhibited IL-6-induced phosphorylation, reduced IL-6 induced STAT3-STAT3 dimerization and nuclear translocation, and reduced cell viability.

Hahm and coworkers[15] reported that Withaferin A suppresses estrogen receptor α expression in human breast cancer cells. Another investigation[16] observed that mitogen-activated protein kinases (MAPK) play a cell line-specific role in the Withaferin A-induced apoptosis of breast cancer cells (MCF-7 and SUM159).

Hahm and coworkers[17] reported that Withaferin A (WA) inhibited oxidative phosphorylation, produced ROS and caused activation of Bak and Bax (promoters of apoptosis) in MCF-7 and MDA-MB-231 cells. They suggested that mitochondria-derived ROS were involved in WA-induced apoptosis.

Hahm and Singh[18] found that Withaferin A treatment of MCF-7, MDA-MB-231, and a spontaneously immortalized, non-tumorogenic normal human epithelial cell line (MCF-10A) induced autophagy. However, induction of autophagy had no effect on lethality in breast cancer cells. Another study[19] reported that Withaferin A-induced apoptosis in breast cancer cells is associated with the suppression of inhibitors of apoptotic family proteins. Withaferin A treatment of MDA-MB-231 and MCF-7 cells downregulated levels of XIAP, cIAP-2 and survivin. However, Withaferin A-mediated inhibition of MDA-MB-231 xenografts in female athymic mice occurred with suppression of survivin without any significant effect on XIAP or cIAP. The authors concluded that "Survivin protein may be a viable biomarker to assess WA exposure and possibly response in human clinical investigation".

Thaiparambil and coworkers[20] reported the antiinvasive and antimetastatic activities of Withaferin A (WA) in breast cancer cells. WA treatment of MDA-MB-231 cells inhibited cell migration, induced perinuclear vimentin accumulation followed by vimentin depolymerization, as well as induced vimentin ser56 phosphorylation. Vimentin is overexpressed in invasive human tumors and is considered a potential molecular target for cancer therapy. The antimetastatic activity of WA was examined using a murine metastatic model. Female BALB/C mice were subcutaneously injected with murine breast carcinoma 4T1 cells into the mammary fat pad. After a week, the mice were treated with the vehicle (i.p.) or WA (i.p.) on alternate days for one month. The WA group showed a decreased rate of tumor growth, tumor weight, tumor proliferation and metastatic lung nodules compared to the vehicle group. Also, primary tumor tissues in the WA group showed increased vimentin ser56 phosphorylation. The authors concluded that "WA is a potent breast cancer antimetastatic agent where its activity at least in part is mediated through its effects on vimentin and vimentin ser56 phosphorylation".

Yang and coworkers[21] reported that a standardized Withania somnifera root extract (SWRE) inhibited cell motility and invasion, as well as disrupted vimentin morphology in breast cancer cells. SWRE was also found to inhibit TGF-β-induced epithelial to mesenchymal transition (EMT) and EMT-induced motility and invasion of human epithelial cells (MCF-10A). The antimetastic efficacy of SWRE was demonstrated using mouse models. BALB/C mice were subcutaneously injected with murine carcinoma 4T1 cells into the mammary fat pad. After one week, the mice were treated with the vehicle (oral gavage), SWRE (1-8 mg/kg/day, oral gavage) or Withaferin A (WA, 1-8 mg/kg/day, i.p.), 3 times per week for 4 weeks. Both the SWRE and WA groups showed a decreased primary tumor volume and number of metastatic lung nodules compared to the vehicle group. In a xenograft mouse model, female athymic nude mice were injected subcutaneously with human metastatic breast cancer cells (MDA-MB-231) into the mammary fat pad. After one week, the mice were treated with the vehicle, SWRE (1-8 mg/

kg/day, oral gavage) or WA (1-8 mg/kg/day, i.p.), 3 times per week for 4 weeks. Both the SWRE and WA groups showed decreased primary tumor volume at the 4 and 8 mg doses, and a decreased number of metastatic lung nodules at the 8 mg dose compared to the vehicle group. The authors pointed out that "these doses of SWRE have nearly no toxicity in normal mouse organs suggesting the potential for clinical use of orally administered WE capsules".

Maliyakkal and coworkers[22] evaluated the cytotoxic and apoptotic activities of aqueous and alcoholic extracts of Withania somnifera root in human breast cancer cells. The aqueous extract did not show significant cytotoxicity in MCF-7 and MDA-MB-231 cells. The ethanol extract showed dose-dependent (1-100 µg/ml) cytotoxicity in both MCF-7 (IC_{50} = 22.33 µg/ml) and MDA-MB-231 (31.99 µg/ml) cells. The cytotoxic effect of the ethanol extract was found to be due to apoptosis and not necrosis.

Zhang and coworkers[23] investigated the anticancer activity of Withaferin A (WA) in MCF-7 breast cancer cells and examined the role of estrogen receptor alpha (ERα) and its associated molecular network. ERα is overexpressed in ER-positive breast cancers. The following observations were made in the treatment of MCF-7 cells with WA compared to controls:

- inhibition of cell growth, decreased cell viability, G2/M cell cycle arrest and induction of apoptosis

- decreased Erα protein levels along with decreased RET tyrosine kinase

- upregulation of phospho-p38 MAPK, p53 and p21

- downregulation of survivin and HSF1

The authors concluded that "WA is a promising agent in cancer therapy".

Kazal and coworkers[24] examined the effect of an alcohol extract of Withania somnifera roots (WSRE) on mammary cancer in rats induced by methylnitrosourea (MNU). MNU-induced carcinoma in rats is similar to estrogen-positive breast cancer in humans. Female Sprague-Dawley rats injected with a single dose of MNU (75 mg/kg, via jugular vein) and treated with WSRE (150 mg/kg/day, via oral gavage) for 155 days showed a 23% reduction in tumor development, 21% reduction in tumor weight and less cell division compared to the group injected with MNU and treated with the vehicle. In a subsequent study, Kazal and coworkers[25] examined the effect of WSRE on ER-negative mammary cancer in mice. Female transgenic

MMTV/Neu mice (52 days old) treated with a diet containing WSRE (750 mg/kg/feed) for 10 months showed a 33% reduction in tumor multiplicity, 10% reduction in tumor weight and less proliferative markers (Ki67 and PCNA) compared to mice treated with a regular diet. Also, Kazal and Hill[26] examined the effect of WSRE on the proliferation and metastasis of MDA-MB-231 breast cancer cells. WSRE treatment of MDA-MB-231 cells reduced cell viability and increased the percentage of cells in the sub-G1 phase. An in vivo experiment demonstrated the antimetastatic effect of WSRE. Athymic Nude-Foxn1[nu] mice (6 weeks old) were injected subcutaneously with MDA-MB-231 cells. After tumors developed (50-200 mm^3), the mice were treated orally with the vehicle (control) or WSRE (300 mg/kg/day) 5 days a week for 8 weeks. The WSRE-treated group showed a reduction in tumor size compared to controls. In the control group, 60% of the mice showed tumor metastasis to the lungs, whereas none in the WSRE group exhibited tumor metastasis.

Hahm and coworkers[27] investigated the efficacy of Withaferin A (WA) in the prevention of breast cancer using a clinically relevant transgenic mouse model. Four-week-old female mouse mammary tumor virus-neu transgenic mice were treated with WA (100 μg, i.p.) or the vehicle three times per week. After 28 weeks, the following observations were made in the WA group compared to the vehicle group: inhibition of tumor progression, reduced incidence of pulmonary metastasis, increased apoptosis and decreased complex III activity, decreased utilization of glucose, decreased glycolysis and reduction of tricarboxylic acid intermediates.

Kim and Singh[28] examined the effect of Withaferin A (WA) on breast cancer stem cells (bCSC) using cellular and in vivo models. WA treatment of MCF-7 (ER-positive) and SUM159 (triple-negative) breast cancer cell lines resulted in fewer mammospheres and a decrease in aldehyde dehydrogenase activity (bCSC biomarkers). The in vivo study showed that the prevention of breast cancer development in MMTV-neu mice by WA treatment was accompanied by fewer mammospheres and decreased aldehyde dehydrogenase activity.

Anthony and coworkers[29] identified β-tubulin as a novel target for Withaferin A (WA) to induce growth arrest in breast cancer cells. Microtubules play a key role in various cellular functions. Treatment of MCF-7, SUM159 and SK-BR-3 cells with WA decreased cell viability, inhibited cell proliferation, arrested cells in the G2/M phase, disrupted the microtubule network and decreased the protein levels of α- and β-tubulin. Withanone (WE) and Withanolide A (WLA) did not show these effects, indicating the importance of the location of the epoxy group for anticancer activity. WA was found to be a superior electrophile compared to WE and WLA by NMR trapping. Mass spectrometric studies showed direct covalent binding of Withaferin A to Cys^{303} of β-tubulin in MCF-7 cells. Docking studies indicated that the WA binding pocket is located on the surface of β-tubulin.

Nagalingam and coworkers[30] explored some anticancer activities of Withaferin A (WA) in breast cancer cells. WA-treated breast cancer cells (MCF-7 and MDA-MB-231) exhibited increased phosphorylation of RSK, ERK and Elk1, and a higher expression of CHOP and DR5. Further experiments revealed that the ERK/RSK signaling axis plays an active role in the regulation and activation of CHOP and Elk1, which contributes to the upregulation of DR5. In vivo studies also showed involvement of the ERK/RSK and CHOP/Elk1 axes, and the role of DR5. The authors concluded that "our results thus demonstrate the integral crosstalk between Withaferin A and ERK/RSK and CHOP/Elk1 axes in breast tumor growth inhibition. Also, our findings may potentially open new avenues of research on the role of Withaferin A as a novel proapoptotic receptor agonist (PARA)".

Lee and coworkers[31] found that Withaferin A inhibited experimental epithelial-mesenchymal transition in MCF-10A cells induced by TNF-α and TGF-β. Also, Withaferin A administration was found to decrease vimentin expression in MDA-MB-231 xenografts as well as in MMTV-neu tumors compared to controls.

Muninathan and coworkers[32] demonstrated that treatment of breast cancer in rats was more effective with paclitaxel along with Withania somnifera compared to paclitaxel or Withania somnifera individually. Female Wistar rats (6-8 weeks old) were treated with 7,12-dimethylbenz(a)anthracene (DMBA, 20 mg in 0.5 ml sunflower oil) three times a week for 28 weeks to induce breast cancer. The cancer-bearing animals were treated with paclitaxel (33 mg/kg) once a week for 4 weeks, Withania somnifera (250 μg) for 30 days or with both paclitaxel and Withania somnifera. Untreated cancer-bearing animals showed a significant increase in lactate dehydrogenase (LDH) compared to controls (animals not treated with DMBA). LDH is the most common enzyme used in cancer patients for prognostic purposes. Cancer bearing animals treated with paclitaxel, Withania somnifera or Withania somnifera+paclitaxel showed decreased LDH compared to untreated cancer-bearing animals. However, the reduction in LDH was much higher in animals of the last group compared to the other two.

10.3 – Colorectal Cancer

The term colorectal cancer is used to describe cancer that starts in the colon and/or rectum. Colon and rectal cancers are grouped together because they share many features. The most commonly diagnosed colon cancer is called adenocarcinoma, which starts in the mucus-secreting glands of the colon. Colorectal cancer is the third most diagnosed cancer in the world, with over 1.8 million new cases estimated to occur in 2018[33].

The treatment for colorectal cancer depends on the size, location and extent to which the cancer has spread. Common treatments include surgery, chemotherapy and radiation. The effect of Withania somnifera on colorectal cancer has been investigated by a number of scientists and the results are summarized below.

Jayaprakasham and coworkers[7] isolated a number of withanolides from Withania somnifera leaves (see Table 10.1) and tested their growth inhibitory activity in HCT-116 colon cancer cells. Most of the compounds inhibited cell growth and Withaferin A was the most active (IC_{50} = 0.30 µg/ml).

Subbaraju and coworkers[8] isolated Ashwagandhanolide from Withania somnifera roots and demonstrated its growth inhibitory activity in HCT-116 cells (IC_{50} = 1.25 µg/ml).

Mulabagal and coworkers[9] showed that Withanolide sulfoxide isolated from the roots of Withania somnifera inhibited the proliferation of HCT-116 cells. In a dose-response study (0.45-7.5 µg/ml), IC_{50} was found to be 3.5 µg/ml.

Siddique and coworkers[34] isolated a withasteroid (5,6-de-epoxy-5-en-7-one-17-hydroxy withaferin A) from the leaves of Withania somnifera and found the compound to be moderately cytotoxic to CACO-2 colon cancer cells (IC_{50} = 3.4 µg/ml).

Koduru and coworkers[35] demonstrated that Withaferin A (WA) inhibited Notch-1 and downregulated prosurvival pathways in colon cancer cells. Treatment of the colon cancer cell lines HCT-116, SW-480 and SW-620 with Withaferin A inhibited cell viability, induced apoptosis, decreased cleaved Notch-1 expression and downregulated its downstream targets, inhibited Akt signaling, and inhibited activation of both IKK-α and IKK-β which reduced the activity of NF-κB. The authors stated that "These results underscore the anticancer activity of WA, which exhibits potential for further development for targeted chemotherapy/prevention strategies in the context of colon cancer".

Suman and coworkers[36] demonstrated by in vivo (xenograft) and in vitro studies that Akt activation induced cell proliferation, angiogenesis and epithelial to mesenchymal transitions in colorectal cells, and Withaferin A was found to inhibit Akt activation and its effects.

Das and coworkers[37] examined the effect of Withaferin A (WA) on the spindle assembly checkpoint (SAC) in colorectal adenocarcinoma cells. SAC is a conserved safety mechanism that functions during mitosis to ensure accurate chromosome distribution between daughter cells. Treatment of HCT-116 and SW480 cells with WA inhibited cell proliferation, increased the accumulation of cells in the G2/M phase and induced apoptosis. In HCT-116 cells, WA caused mitotic delay by blocking SAC function and causing chromosomal abnormality. Treatment of HCT-116 and SW480 cells with WA decreased the levels of Mad2-Cdc20 (important constituents of the SAC complex). It was found that WA induced proteasomal degradation of the Mad2-Cdc20 complex in these cells and lowered its steady-state level. The authors hypothesized that "Withaferin A kills cancer cells by delaying the mitotic exit followed by inducing chromosomal instability".

Choi and Kim[38] examined the anticancer effect of Withaferin A (WA) in vitro and in vivo against human colorectal cancer. WA treatment of HCT-116 cells decreased the viability of cells and reduced cell migration. WA treatment of HCT-116 cells incubated with IL-6 inhibited IL-6 induced STAT3 reporter gene activity. The in vivo study was conducted using a xenograft mouse model. BALB/C nude mice (6 week-old) were subcutaneously injected with HCT-116 cells and after 7 days were randomized into two groups. One group served as a control. The other group was treated with WA (2 mg/kg, i.p.) on alternate days for 32 days. The WA group showed reduced tumor volume and weight, as well as inhibition of PCNA expression (a marker of tumor cell proliferation) compared to the control group.

Muralikrishnan and coworkers[39] reported that Withania somnifera altered the levels of leucocytes, lymphocytes, immune complexes and immunoglobulins (Ig) A, G, and M in azoxymethane-induced colon cancer in mice. Another study[40] observed a decrease in tricarboxylic acid enzymes such as ICDH, SDH, MDH and α-KGDH in azoxymethane-induced colon cancer in mice. Administering Withania somnifera reversed these changes to control levels. The authors suggested that "W. somnifera is the promising chemotherapeutic agent for the treatment of colon cancer".

10.4 – Cervical Cancer

Cervical cancer is a type of cancer that starts in the cervix, the lower part of the uterus. Most cervical cancers are caused by persistent infection with a high-risk type of human papillomavirus (HPV) such as HPV-16 or HPV-18. The two main types of cervical cancer are squamous cell carcinoma and adenocarcinoma. Squamous cell carcinoma, which accounts for about 90% of all cervical cancers, develops from cells in the exocervix and the cancer cells have features of squamous cells. Cervical adenocarcinoma develops from the mucus-producing gland cells of the endocervix.

Cervical cancer is the fourth most commonly diagnosed cancer in women worldwide. About 570,000 new cases of cervical cancer and 300,000 deaths due to cervical cancer were estimated to occur in 2018. Approximately 80% of cervical cancer cases and 85% of cervical cancer-related deaths occur in low and middle-income countries. The death rates of cervical cancer have reduced by 75% in the developed world[41,42].

Cervical cancer is treated with surgery, radiation, chemotherapy or a combination of the three. A number of investigators have studied the effect of Withania somnifera on cervical cancer and some of the published results are summarized below.

Munagala and coworkers[43] examined the effect of Withaferin A (WA) on human cervical cancer cells. WA treatment of the cervical cancer cell lines C33a, CaSki, HeLa and SiHa inhibited cell growth in a dose-dependent manner. The IC_{50} values were 0.2, 0.45, 1.0 and 1.2 µM for C33a, CaSki, HeLa and SiHa respectively. In HPV-positive cells (CaSki, HeLa and SiHa), WA downregulated HPV E6 oncoprotein expression and increased p53 (tumor suppressor protein) and $p21^{cip/waf1}$. In HPV-negative cells, only $p21^{cip1/waf1}$ increased. WA treatment of CaSki cells caused G2/M phase cell arrest, decreased the level of STAT3 and its phosphorylation, decreased Bcl-2, increased Bax, and induced PARP cleavage and caspase 3 activity. An in vivo study was done using a xenograft mouse model. Female athymic nu/nu mice (5-6 weeks-old) were injected with CaSki Cells into the right flank and the next day they were divided into two groups. One group was treated with the vehicle and other with WA (8 mg/kg, i.p.) on alternate days for 6 weeks. The WA-treated group showed a reduction in tumor growth compared to controls. Some of the other WA-induced changes observed in the vitro study were also seen in the vivo study. The authors stated that "Together our data suggest that WA can be exploited as a potent therapeutic agent for the treatment and prevention of cervical cancer without deleterious effects".

Cui and coworkers[44] demonstrated that Withaferin A enhanced hyperthermia-induced apoptosis in human cervical cancer HeLa cells, and this was accompanied by intracellular ROS generation and a decreased GSH/GSSG ratio. Treatment of HeLa cells with WA (1.0 µM) or hyperthermia (44 °C) alone had no significant effect on mitochondrial transmembrane potential (MMP), an index of mitochondrial function. WA + hyperthermia increased MMP, increased proapoptotic and decreased antiapoptotic Bcl-2 family proteins, and increased expression of cleaved caspase-3. The authors stated that "WA enhances hyperthermia-induced apoptosis via a mitochondria-caspase dependent pathaway; its underlying mechanism involves elevated intracellular oxidative stress, mitochondria dysfunction, and JNK activation".

Lee and coworkers[45] reported that Withaferin A (WA) treatment of CaSki cells inhibited TGF-β-induced metalloproteinase (MMP)-9 activity and MMP-9 mRNA, reduced invasiveness and inhibited phosphorylation of Akt. Also, WA treatment of CaSki cells inhibited PMA-induced MMP-9 activity and MMP-9 mRNA. The authors concluded that "These findings indicate that use of Withaferin A may be an effective strategy for control of metastasis and invasiveness of tumors".

Kim[46] reported that Withaferin A treatment of CaSki cells inhibited PMA induced MMP-9 activity and MMP-9 mRNA, decreased NF-κB activity and suppressed cell migration. The authors concluded that "our findings suggest that withaferin A might inhibit PMA-induced migration through downregulation of MMP-9 expression and activity".

Jha and coworkers[47] showed that treatment of HeLa cells with an alcohol extract of Withania somnifera roots inhibited cell viability, induced apoptosis and reversed the hypermethylation of retinoic acid receptor β2 (RARβ2). RARβ2 is a putative tumor suppressor gene and its expression is reduced in various cancers by methylation.

Ye and Song[48] found that Withaferin A treatment of HeLa cells decreased cell viability and suppressed the expression of antiapoptotic genes.

Kumar and coworkers[49] examined in silico the binding interaction of 12 plant-originated ligands including Withaferin A with oncoproteins E6 and E7 of HPV-16 and HPV-18. All 12 plant ligands were found to bind with HPV oncoproteins, but Withaferin A was the most effective. The authors suggested that "Withaferin A may be used as a common drug for cervical cancer caused by high risk HPV types, perhaps by restoring normal functions of tumor suppressor proteins".

10.5 – Prostate Cancer

Worldwide, prostate cancer is the second most common cancer in men, with an estimated 1.3 million new cases in 2018[50]. Prostate cancer develops in the prostate, a part of the male reproductive system located just below the bladder and in front of the rectum. It surrounds the upper part of the urethra, the tube that empties urine from the bladder. The prostate secretes fluid that nourishes and protects sperm. There are many types of prostate cancer, with adenocarcinomas being the most common.

Treatments for prostate cancer include surgery, chemotherapy, radiation therapy and hormone therapy. A number of investigators have examined the effect of Withania somnifera on prostate cancer and some results are summarized below.

Srinivasan and coworkers[51] found that Withaferin A (WA) induced apoptosis in androgen-refractory prostate cancer cells (PC-3). In androgen-responsive prostate cancer cells (LNCaP), neither WA nor the antiandrogens flutamide or Casodex individually induced apoptosis. However, WA in combination with either antiandrogen induced apoptosis. The mechanism of apoptosis in PC-3 cells was found to involve induction of the prostate apoptotic response 4 (Par-4) gene, activation of caspases, inhibition of NF-κB and downregulation of Bcl-2 expression. An in vivo study was conducted by using a xenograft mouse model. PC-3 cells were injected into nude (nu/nu) mice (5-6 weeks old) and tumors were allowed to grow. These mice were given the vehicle or WA (5 mg/kg) intratumorally 5 days a week for 4 weeks. The vehicle group showed continuous tumor growth, whereas the WA group showed inhibition of tumor growth. The tumors from the WA group showed Par-4 upregulation and apoptosis.

Roy and coworkers[52] examined the cell cycle regulatory potential of Withaferin A (WA) in prostate cancer cell lines. Treatment of PC-3 and DU-145 cells with WA decreased cell viability and induced G2/M cell cycle arrest accompanied by upregulation of p21 and downregulation of the cyclins E2, A2 and B1. WA treatment of PC-3 cells activated Wee-1, induced Aurora B expression and inhibited microtubule polymerization. Prostate tumors express very low levels of Wee-1, which has been recognized as a useful therapeutic target for prostate cancer. The authors concluded that "the results reported herein demonstrate that Withaferin A induces cell cycle arrest at the

G2/M phase and this arrest may inhibit the growth of prostate cancer cells".

Nishikawa and coworkers[53] examined the effects of Withaferin A (WA) on the androgen-independent prostate cancer cell lines PC-3 and DU-145, the androgen-responsive prostate cancer cell line (LNCaP), and normal human fibroblasts (TIG-1 and KD). WA induced cell death in PC-3 and DU-145. LNCaP, TIG-1 and KD showed resistance to WA.

Rao and coworkers[54] evaluated the effect of alcoholic extracts of 13 different plants on prostate cancer cell lines with differing metastatic potential. Out of the 13 extracts, Withania somnifera, C. longa and P. cuspidatum inhibited colony formation in PC-3M (highly metastatic), DU-145 (moderately metastatic) and LNCaP (poorly metastatic) cells even at low concentrations. The authors suggested that "these three agents have good potential for further studies against prostate cancer cell lines".

Aalinkeel and coworkers[55] found that treating PC-3 cells with an alcohol extract of Withania somnifera roots inhibited cell growth, downregulated gene and protein expression of the proinflammatory cytokines IL-6, IL-1β, Chemokine IL-8, Hsp70 and STAT-2, and upregulated the gene and protein expression of p38 MAPK, PI3K, caspase-6, Cyclin D and c-myc. Extract treatment also modulated the JAK-STAT pathway.

Yadav and coworkers[56] showed that ethanol (50%) extracts of Withania somnifera roots, stems and leaves were cytotoxic to PC-3 and DU-145 cells.

Singh and coworkers[57] reported that Withaferin A inhibited prostate tumor growth by potentiating an antitumor immune response.

10.6 – Lung Cancer

Lung cancer is the most commonly occurring cancer in men and the third most commonly occurring cancer in women worldwide, with an estimated 2 million new cases in 2018[58]. Lung cancer develops in the lungs and has two major types: small cell lung cancer and non-small cell lung cancer. Small cell lung cancer comprises about 10-15% and occurs in heavy smokers. Non-small cell lung cancer accounts for about 85% and includes squamous cell carcinoma, adenocarcinoma and large cell carcinoma.

The most commonly used treatments for lung cancer include surgery, radiation therapy, chemotherapy and targeted therapy. A number of investigators have examined the effect of Withania somnifera on lung cancer and some of the results are summarized below.

Jayaprakasam and coworkers[7] isolated twelve withanolides from Withania somnifera leaves (see Table 10.1). These compounds and diacetyl withaferin A were tested for their antiproliferative activity in NCI-H460 lung cancer cells. Most of the compounds inhibited cell growth. Withaferin A showed the greatest antiproliferation effect (IC_{50} = 0.24 μg/ml).

Subbaraju and coworkers[8] isolated Ashwagandhanolide, a dimeric thiowithanolide, from the roots of Withania somnifera and demonstrated its growth-inhibiting activity against the lung cancer cell line NCI-H460.

Chowdhary and coworkers[59] isolated a chlorinated steroidal lactone, a diepoxy withanolide and Withaferin A from the aerial parts of Withania somnifera and tested their cytotoxic activity against the human lung cancer cell line NCI-H460. All three compounds inhibited cell growth. Withaferin A was the most effective (IC_{50} = 0.18 μg/ml, LC_{50} = 0.45 μg/ml).

Singh and coworkers[60] examined the effect of Withania somnifera (WS) on urethane-induced lung adenomas in mice. Administration of urethane (125 mg/kg, S.C.) to adult male albino mice twice a week for 7 months induced lung adenomas, decreased body weight, increased mortality and decreased lymphocytes. Administration of WS (200 mg/kg/day, P.O.) along with urethane protected the animals from developing tumors and reversed the other changes induced by urethane. The authors noted that "W. somnifera may be preventing urethane induced lung adenomas by inducing a state of non specific increase in resistance (adaptogen) and immunostimulant properties".

Neema and coworkers[61] found that a hydroalcoholic extract of Withania somnifera leaves was cytotoxic to the lung cancer cell line A549 (IC_{50} = 11 μg/ml).

Senthilnathan and coworkers[62] examined the chemotherapeutic efficacy of Paclitaxel (antineoplastic agent) along with an alcoholic extract of Withania somnifera roots (WS) on benzo(a)pyrene-induced lung cancer in mice. Adult male Swiss albino mice were treated with benzo(a)pyrene (50 mg/kg, P.O.) dissolved in corn oil, twice a week for 4 weeks to induce lung cancer. After 12 weeks of cancer induction, the animals were treated with corn oil, paclitaxel (33 mg/kg/day, i.p.) or paclitaxel (33 mg/kg/day, i.p.) + WS (400 mg/kg/day, P.O.) for 4 weeks. Normal mice treated with corn oil served as controls. Cancer-bearing mice treated with corn oil showed decreased body weight, increased lung weight, increased activities of tumor marker enzymes (aryl hydrocarbon hydroxylase, γ–glutamyl transpeptidase, 5'-nucleotidase and lactate dehydrogenase) in the lungs and serum, and increased levels of glycoproteins (hexose, hexosamine and sialic acid) and polyamines in the lungs compared to controls. Cancer-bearing animals treated with paclitaxel or paclitaxel+WS showed a reversal of these changes. The paclitaxel+WS treatment was more effective than paclitaxel alone. Another investigation[63] found that WS enhanced the effect of paclitaxel in stabilizing ATPase enzymes and decreasing lipid peroxidation in cancer-bearing animals. Senthilinathan and coworkers[64] also showed that Withania somnifera enhanced the effect of paclitaxel on tricarboxylic acid cycle key enzymes and electron transport chain complexes in benzo(a)pyrene treated mice.

Yong and coworkers[65] examined the anticancer effect of Withaferin A in non-small cell lung cancer (NSCLC). Treatment of the NSCLC cell line A549 with Withaferin A inhibited cell proliferation, induced apoptosis, increased levels of cleaved caspase-3 and decreased Bcl-2 and p-Akt/Akt.

Liu and coworkers[66] also reported the anticancer effect of Withaferin A in NSCLC A549 cells. Treatment of A549 cells with Withaferin A (0-50 µM) caused loss of cell viability (IC_{50} = 10 µM, 24 h), induced apoptosis, caused loss of mitochondrial membrane potential, activated caspase-3 and caspase-9, and produced ROS. A549 cells treated with Withaferin A and incubated with N-acetyl cysteine (NAC) showed a reversal of the changes observed in the absence of NAC. This indicates the importance of ROS in the cytotoxicity of WA on A549 cells.

10.7 – Fibrosarcoma

Fibrosarcoma is a rare type of cancer. It originates in fibroblast cells that produce connective tissues throughout the body. Fibrosarcoma tumors can develop anywhere, but are frequently found in the legs, arms and pelvis. Treatments for fibrosarcoma include surgery, chemotherapy and radiation. A few investigations have examined the effect of Withania somnifera on fibrosarcoma and the results are summarized below.

Prakash and coworkers[67] investigated the chemopreventive ability of a Withania somnifera root extract (WSE) against 20-methylcholanthrene (MCA)-induced fibrosarcoma tumors in mice. Swiss albino mice were given a single dose of DMSO (0.1 ml, S.C.), a single dose of MCA (200 mg/0.1 ml DMSO, S.C.) or treated with WSE (400 mg/kg/day, P.O.) for one week followed by a single dose of MCA and further treatment with WSE for 15 weeks. The DMSO group showed no fibrosarcoma and a 100% survival rate. The MCA group showed earlier tumor appearance, more tumors, larger tumors and shorter lifespans compared to the WSE+MCA group. Also, liver tissue homogenate of the MCA group showed increased LPO and decreased GSH, SOD, CAT and GST compared to the DMSO and WSE+MCA groups. The authors concluded that "it seems probable that WSE can be used as an adjuvant to local tumor excision and may increase overall survival rate, however more experimental and clinical data is required to support this statement". Davis and Kuttan[68] also reported similar results in an earlier investigation.

Kaileh and coworkers[69] reported that Withania somnifera was cytotoxic to murine fibrosarcoma L929sA cells.

Widodo and coworkers[70] examined the effect of an Ashwagandha leaf extract on fibrosarcoma tumors in mice. A methanol extract of Ashwagandha leaves was extracted with hexane and then with ether. The ether extract was dried and dissolved in DMSO for the study. BALB/C nude mice injected subcutaneously with HT1080 cells developed tumors after 10-15 days. When these mice were treated with the extract either before or after the formation of tumor buds, tumor growth was suppressed. Withanone was identified as the component in the extract responsible for tumor growth suppression. A subsequent investigation[71] identified different pathways by which the extract kills cancer. These pathways include p53 signaling, GM-CFS signaling, death receptor signaling, apoptosis signaling and the G2-M DNA damage regulation pathway.

10.8 – Neuroblastoma

Neuroblastoma is a type of cancer that starts in the tissues of the sympathetic nervous system. Neuroblastoma commonly begins in the nerve tissue of the adrenal glands, but may also develop in other areas including the chest, neck and spine. Neuroblastoma is most commonly diagnosed in children under the age of 5. About 800 new cases of neuroblastoma are diagnosed each year in the United States[72]. The effect of Withania somnifera on neuroblastoma cells has been studied by a few investigators and the results are summarized below.

Kataria and coworkers[73] investigated the anticancer activity of an aqueous extract of Withania somnifera leaves (ASH-WEX) against neuroblastoma cell lines. ASH-WEX treatment of human neuroblastoma cell lines IMR-32, TGW and SH-SY5Y, and mouse neuroblastoma cell line Neuro-2a inhibited cell proliferation. In IMR-32, ASH-WEX treatment resulted in the following observations:

- morphological changes as well as increased NF200, HSP 70, mortalin and Akt-P expression, indicating the induction of cell differentiation

- decreased expression of cyclin D1 and the antiapoptotic marker Bcl-xl

- increased percentage of cells in the G0/G1 phase

- increased expression of neural cell adhesion molecule (NCAM) and decreased expression of its polysialylated form (PSA-NCAM)

- decreased MMP-2 and MMP-9

The authors concluded that "the current study supports the idea that ASH-WEX may have the potential to reduce the malignancy of neuroblastomas".

Yco and coworkers[74] examined the effect of Withaferin A (WA) on human neuroblastoma (NB) cell lines. WA treatment of the human NB cell lines Be(2)-c, SMS-KCNR, SH-SY5Y, IMR-32 and LAN-5 induced cell death. WA suppressed STAT-3 Phosphorylation. Computational modeling and docking simulations showed that WA binds STAT3 near the Y705 phosphotyrosine residue similarly to BP-1-102, a potent STAT3 inhibitor.

10.9 – Skin Cancer

Skin cancer begins in the epidermis (outer skin layer), which has three types of cells: basal cells, squamous cells and melanocytes. Correspondingly, there are three major forms of skin cancer: basal cell carcinoma, squamous cell carcinoma and melanoma. Each year, two to three million non-melanoma and 132,000 melanoma cancer cases occur globally[75]. Basal cell carcinoma is the most common cancer. There are many treatments for skin cancer including surgery, radiation therapy and chemotherapy. A number of studies have been conducted to understand the effect of Withania somnifera on skin cancer and the results are summarized below.

Davis and Kuttan[76] examined the effect of a methanol (70%) extract of Withania somnifera roots (WS) on 7,12-dimethylbenzanthracene (DMBA)-induced carcinogenesis in mice. Swiss albino mice were treated with WS (20 mg/kg/day, i.p.) for 5 days followed by a single topical application of DMBA. WS treatment was continued twice a week for 10 weeks. Croton oil was applied topically two weeks after initiation, twice a week for 6 weeks. The control group was prepared similarly, except the animals were not treated with WS. The WS group showed fewer tumors compared to the control group. Also, the WS group showed increased levels of GSH (liver and skin), GST (liver and skin), GPx (liver) and CAT (liver), and decreased LPO (liver) compared to the control group.

Prakash and coworkers[77] also reported that a hydroalcoholic extract of Withania somnifera roots prevented DMBA-induced squamous cell carcinoma in Swiss alibino mice. They suggested that "The chemopreventive activity may be linked to the antioxidant/free radical scavenging constituents of the extract".

Padmavathi and coworkers[78] showed that a diet containing Withania somnifera roots reduced DMBA-induced tumor incidence in Swiss albino mice.

Leyon and Kuttan[79] studied the effect of a methanol (70%) extract of Withania somnifera roots (WS) and withanolide D on B16F-10 melanoma-induced metastasis in mice. Male C57BL mice were given a single injection of B16F-10 (via lateral tail vein) and treated with WS (20 mg, i.p.) or withanolide D (500 μg) once per day for 10 days. The control group received a single injection of B16F-10 and was treated with the vehicle. Groups treated with WS and withanolide D showed inhibition of metastatic colony formation in the lungs, increased life span, decreased levels of hydroxyproline, uronic acid and hexosamine in the lungs, and decreased levels of serum sialic acid and γ-GT compared to the control group.

Mathur and coworkers[80] examined the effect of 1-oxo-5β,6β-epoxy-witha-2-enolide (WSC) isolated from Withania somnifera roots on skin carcinoma in rats. Carcinoma was induced in male Wistar rats by exposing a shaved portion of dorsal skin to UV B radiation (294 nm, $4 \times 10^4 J/m^2/s$) one hour per day for 20 days. Some of these rats were additionally treated with a topical application of benzoyl peroxide (20 mg/0.2 ml of acetone) twice a week for one month. In the radiation-only rats, microsections of irradiated skin tissue showed malignant cells in the epidermal region and distinct clusters of cells with p53+ foci (measure of tumor risk). In the radiation+benzoyl peroxide rats, microsections of irradiated skin showed an epidermis of varying thickness with premalignant cells and p53+ foci. Some rats were treated with WSC (20 mg/kg/day) for 5 days before exposure to radiation, and during the 20-day radiation treatment they were pretreated with WSC 30 minutes before radiation exposure. These rats showed no malignant cells or p53+ foci in the epidermis of exposed skin. Also, rats treated with radiation followed by benzoyl peroxide and then WSC showed no malignancy or p53+ foci in microsections of irradiated skin. The authors concluded that "These results prove that 1-oxo-5β,6β-epoxy-witha-2-enolide has the potential for acting as an agent to prevent incidence of skin carcinoma induced by UV B radiation".

Mayola and coworkers[81] investigated the effects of Withaferin A (WA) on a number of human melanoma cells. WA treatment of the human cutaneous melanoma cell lines Lu1205, M14, Mel501 and SK28 reduced cell viability, induced apoptosis, increased generation of intracellular ROS, caused loss of transmembrane potential ($\Delta\Psi$m), released proapoptotic cytochrome C from the mitochondrial intermembrane space to the cytosol, and activated caspase-3 and caspase-9. Also, the ratios of Bcl-2/Bax and Bcl-2/Bim decreased, indicating proapoptotic potential. The authors concluded that "Altogether, these results support the therapeutic potential of WA against human melanoma".

Halder and coworkers[82] showed that treating malignant melanoma A375 cells with an aqueous extract of Withania somnifera roots reduced cell viability, induced morphological changes, induced nuclear blebbing and apoptotic bodies, and caused DNA fragmentation.

Uma Devi and coworkers[83] examined the radiosensitizing effect of Withaferin A on B16F1 mouse melanoma cells. C57BL mice were injected intradermally on the dorsal skin with B16F1 cells. After the development of tumors, the animals were treated with WA (10-60 mg/kg, i.p.) or WA followed by local tumor irradiation (30 Gy). One group of tumor-bearing animals was treated with the vehicle followed by local tumor irradiation. The animals were observed for 120 days. Groups treated with WA, WA+irradiation or vehicle+irradiation showed increased tumor volume doubling time (VDT) and growth delay time (GD) compared to the vehicle-only treated group. The WA+irradiation group showed significantly higher VDT and GD than the other groups. The authors concluded that "The present results indicate that the radiation response of this tumor can be significantly enhanced by pretreatment with withaferin A".

Uma Devi and Kamath[84] investigated the radiosensitizing effect of Withaferin A (WA) in combination with acute and fractionated radiotherapy (RT) and hyperthermia (HT). C57BL mice bearing B16F1 melanoma were treated by a single modality (WA, RT or HT), bimodality (WA+RT, WA+HT or RT+HT), or trimodality (WA+RT+HT). The animals were observed for 120 days and VDT, GD and % regression with no growth were measured. The trimodality treatment with fractionated RT was the most effective. The authors concluded that "Withaferin A seems to be a promising radiosensitizer for use with radiotherapy of radioresistant solid tumors. However, more work is needed to establish a safe drug dose for administration with conventional radiation dose fractions in humans". A later investigation[85] found that "WA is a better radio-sensitizer than HT in fractionated regimen and the response of radioresistant tumors like melanoma can be significantly enhanced by combining nontoxic doses of WA with fractionated RT, with or without HT, allowing decrease in radiation dose.

Kalthur and coworkers[86] examined the effect of Withaferin A (WA) on the development and decay of thermotolerance in B16F1 melanoma in C57BL mice. Tumors were subjected to HT (43 °C, 30 min) followed by WA (40 mg, i.p.). Tumors were then subjected to a second HT after specified time intervals. The control group received similar treatment, except carboxymethyl cellulose was injected instead of WA. The WA group showed increased GD values with an increased time gap between two hyperthermia treatments compared to the corresponding numbers in the control group.

Li and Zhao[87] reported that Withaferin A suppressed tumor promoter 12-O-tetradecanoylphorbol 13- acetate-induced cell transformation and proliferation in murine skin epidermal JB6 Cl-41 P+ cells. In another study, Li and coworkers[88] demonstrated the chemopreventive potential of Withaferin A using a chemically induced skin carcinogenesis mouse model. Withaferin A suppressed skin tumor formation by suppressing cell proliferation and not by inducing apoptosis during skin carcinogenesis. Also, Withaferin A blocked carcinogen-induced upregulation of acetyl-CoA carboxylase.

10.10 – Ovarian Cancer

Ovarian cancer starts in the ovary's (female reproductive system) germ, stromal or epithelial cells. Epithelial carcinoma makes up about 90% of ovarian cancer[89]. Surgery and chemotherapy are generally used to treat ovarian cancer. A number of studies have been conducted to understand the effect of Withania somnifera on ovarian cancer and the results are summarized below.

Zhang and coworkers[90] examined the effect of Withaferin A (WA) on ovarian cancer cells. WA treatment of the ovarian cancer cell lines CaOV3, SKOV3, OVCAR3, TOV112D and TOV21G inhibited cell viability. In CaOV3 and SKOV3 cells, WA inhibited colony formation, induced apoptosis, increased PARP cleavage, decreased pro-caspase-3, caused G2/M phase cell cycle arrest and decreased protein levels of cdc25C. WA decreased Notch3 protein levels in CaOV3 cells and Notch1 protein levels in SKO3 cells.

Kakar and coworkers[91] found that Withaferin A (WA) in combination with low doses of cisplatin exerted a synergistic cytotoxic effect on ovarian cancer cells. Cisplatin is frequently used in the treatment of ovarian cancer. It is fairly effective in high doses but causes serious side effects. Treatment of the ovarian cancer cell lines A2780, CAOV3 and A2780/CP70 with WA, cisplatin or WA+cisplatin induced cell death. WA+cisplatin was more effective than WA or cisplatin alone. A smaller amount of cisplatin with WA produced the same effect as a larger amount of cisplatin alone. Treatment of cells with cisplatin (20 µM) produced no morphological changes; treatment with WA (1.5 µM) produced moderate morphological changes; treatment with cisplatin (20 µM) + WA (1.5 µM) produced significant morphological changes characteristic of apoptosis. Treatment of A2780 cells with WA (0.5 µM) + cisplatin (20 µM) was more effective in producing ROS and causing DNA damage than WA or cisplatin alone. It is evident that low doses of cisplatin along with WA produce the same effects as high doses of cisplatin alone, without causing adverse side effects. In a subsequent investigation, Kakar and coworkers[92] examined the effect of Withaferin A (WA), cisplatin (CIS) and WA+CIS on tumor growth and metastasis on nude mice bearing orthotopic ovarian cancer. A2780 cancer cells were injected into the left ovary of nu/nu female mice (5-6 weeks old). Ten days later, the animals were treated with the vehicle (control group), WA (2 mg/kg, i.p., every other day), CIS (6 mg/kg, i.p., once a week) or WA+CIS for 4 weeks. The control group showed large tumors and metastasis to the right ovary, liver and lungs. Animals treated with WA, CIS or WA+CIS showed decreased tumor weight compared to the control group and no metastasis. Treatment with WA+CIS was more effective than WA or CIS alone. The authors suggested that "WA alone or in combination with CIS may serve as a safer and more efficacious therapy for both first line and second line options for ovarian cancer".

Fong and coworkers[93] showed that Withaferin A (WA) synergistically enhanced the anticancer activity of doxorubicin (DOX) against ovarian cancer cells. Treatment of the ovarian cancer cell lines A2780, A2780/CP70 and CaOV3 with WA, DOX or WA+DOX inhibited cell proliferation, increased ROS generation and induced cell death. WA+DOX was more effective than WA or DOX alone. WA (1.5 and 2 µM)-treated cells showed a few autophagosomes and intact mitochondria. DOX (200 µM)-treated cells showed autophagosomes containing cytoplasm and destruction of mitochondria. DOX (200 µM) + WA (2 µM)-treated cells showed intense autophagic vacuoles and an absence of mitochondria, indicating intense cell damage. The antitumor efficacy of WA+DOX was also demonstrated by using minitumor and xenograft models. The authors suggested that "combining low dose of DOX with suboptimal dose of WA can serve as a potential therapy for the treatment of ovarian cancer with potential to minimize/eliminate the side effects associated with higher doses of DOX".

Barua and coworkers[94] investigated the effect of dietary Ashwagandha (ASH) supplementation on ovarian tumors in laying hens. White Leghorn laying hens (3-4 years old) were fed a basal ration (control group) or a basal ration supplemented with 1% or 2% Ashwagandha root powder for 90 days. Each group had 25 hens with normal ovaries and 5 with ovarian tumors (early stage). In the control group, all five cancer-bearing hens progressed to late stage cancer with metastasis, whereas in the 1% and 2% ASH groups the corresponding numbers were 4 and 1 respectively. Among all normal hens, 4 in the control group, 2 in the 1% ASH group and 1 in the 2% ASH group developed early stage ovarian tumors confined to the ovary. Ashwagandha treatment of cancer-bearing hens showed an increased population of stromal and tumor-infiltrating NK cells, and a decreased expression of MICA. The authors concluded that "This study may be useful for clinical study to determine the effects of dietary Ashwagandha on NK cell immune function in patients with ovarian cancer".

10.11 – Pancreatic Cancer

Pancreatic cancer is an aggressive type of cancer that develops in the tissues of the pancreas. There are two main types of pancreatic cancer: exocrine and endocrine. About 94% of pancreatic cancers are exocrine tumors[95]. They develop in exocrine cells that produce digestive enzymes. About 6% of pancreatic cancers are endocrine tumors. They develop in endocrine cells that produce insulin and other hormones.

Treatments for pancreatic cancer include surgery, chemotherapy and radiation therapy. The effect of Withania somnifera on pancreatic cancer has been studied by a number scientists and the results are summarized below.

Yu and coworkers[96] examined the efficacy of Withaferin A (WA) against pancreatic cancer. WA inhibited cell proliferation in the human pancreatic cancer cell lines Panc-1, BxPc3 and MiaPaCa-2. In Panc-1 cells, WA induced apoptosis, inhibited Hsp90 chaperone activity and induced Hsp90 client protein degradation. WA was found to bind directly to Hsp90 and Hsp90 degradation was proteasome-dependent. Also, WA disrupted the Hsp90-Cdc37 complex. In vivo studies using a pancreatic xenograft mouse model showed that WA treatment of mice bearing Panc-1 tumors inhibited tumor growth. The authors concluded that "These data provide a potential of Withaferin A as a novel Hsp90 inhibitor for use against pancreatic cancers".

Grover and coworkers[97] showed by docking studies that Withaferin A has the potential to inhibit the association of the chaperone Hsp90 to its co-chaperone Cdc37 by disrupting the attachment of Hsp90 to Cdc37. The authors suggested that "Withaferin A is a potent anticancer agent as ascertained by its potent Hsp90-client modulating capability".

Li and coworkers[98] demonstrated the synergistic antitumor activity of Withaferin A (WA) with oxaliplatin against human pancreatic cells. Oxaliplatin is effective in high doses but has severe side effects. Treatment of the human pancreatic cells Panc-1, MIAPaCa-2 and SW1990 with WA, oxaliplatin or WA+oxaliplatin inhibited cell growth. WA+oxaliplatin was more effective than WA or oxaliplatin alone. The greatest synergistic effect was observed with Panc-1 and MIAPaC-2. Treatment of these cell lines with WA (2 µM) + oxaliplatin (25 µM) induced caspase-dependent apoptosis. The mechanism of apoptosis was found to involve generation of ROS, mitochondrial dysfunction and inhibition of PI3K/AKT signaling. In vivo studies using a xenograft model gave similar results. The authors concluded that "combination therapy of oxaliplatin and WA could become a novel approach for PC treatment. Clinical trials must be exploited to support this strategy for PC treatment".

Sarkar and coworkers[99] found that Withanolide D treatment of the pancreatic cancer cell lines MIAPaCa2, AsPC1, Panc10.05, Panc1 and BxPC3 inhibited cell proliferation. Treatment of MIAPaCa2 cells with Withanolide D decreased cell viability, increased the number of TUNEL-positive cells, decreased the ratio of Bcl-2 (antiapoptotic) to Bax (proapoptotic), increased the activation of caspase 8 and caspase 3, increased the accumulation of cells in the G2/M phase, and upregulated Chk1 and Chk 2. The authors concluded that "this finding suggests the potential identification of a new lead molecule in the treatment of pancreatic adenocarcinoma".

10.12 – Blood cancer

Blood cancer begins in blood-forming tissues or in the cells of the immune system. The three main groups of blood cancer are leukemia, lymphoma and myeloma. Leukemia originates in blood-forming tissues, lymphoma forms in lymphocytes, and myeloma begins in blood plasma cells. Treatments for blood cancer include chemotherapy, radiation therapy and stem cell transplantation. A number of investigators have examined the effect of Withania somnifera on blood cancer and the results are summarized below.

Senthil and coworkers[100] examined the anticancer effect of a methanol extract of Withania somnifera leaves and a withanolide isolated from the extract. Treatment of HL-60 leukemia cells with the extract or withanolide inhibited cell proliferation, induced apoptosis, upregulated Bax, downregulated Bcl-2, caused loss of mitochondrial membrane potential, released cytochrome c into the cytosol, and increased the activities of caspase 8, caspase 9 and caspase 3.

Malik and coworkers[101] examined the anticancer activity of Withaferin A against HL-60 human myeloid leukemia cells. The following observations were made about the treatment of HL-60 cells with Withaferin A:

- inhibition of cell proliferation
- induction of apoptosis
- generation of ROS
- loss of mitochondrial membrane potential
- cleavage of PARP and activation of caspase 3, caspase 8 and caspase 9
- increase of Bax expression in the mitochondrial fraction along with an increase of cytochrome release from mitochondria to the cytosol
- decreased Bid expression
- translocation of apoptosis-inducing factor from mitochondrial intermembrane space to nuclei
- inhibition of NF-κB activation

Pretreating HL-60 cells with N-acetyl cysteine attenuated the effects of Withaferin A treatment. The authors concluded that "The results of our studies demonstrate that Withaferin A-induced early ROS generation and mitochondrial dysfunction in cancer cells trigger events responsible for mitochondrial-dependent and -independent apoptosis pathways".

Mandal and coworkers[102] showed that Withaferin A (WA) inhibited cell growth in several types of leukemic cells and primary cells from patients with lymphoblastic and myeloid leukemia. WA showed no such effect in normal human lymphocytes. Treatment of MOLT-4 cells with WA induced apoptosis, increased the accumulation of cells in the sub-G0 phase, increased Bax expression (proapoptotic) and the Bax/Bcl-2 ratio, decreased mitochondrial transmembrane potential, released cytochrome c from mitochondria to the cytosol, activated caspase 3 and caspase 9, induced PARP cleavage and activated p38MAPK. The authors concluded that Withaferin A "holds promise as a new, potential, alternative inexpensive chemotherapeutic agent for the treatment of patients with leukemia of both lymphoid and myeloid origin". In a subsequent investigation, Mondal and coworkers[103] demonstrated the anticancer activity of Withanolide D against lymphoid (MOLT-4), myeloid (K562), and fresh leukemia cells from patients. Treatment of MOLT-4 and K562 cells with Withanolide D inhibited cell growth, induced apoptosis, increased ceramide production and increased JNK and p38MAPK phosphorylation. Ceramide accumulation was found to be the result of sphingomyelin hydrolysis. Similar observations were made with fresh leukemia cells treated with Withanolide D. The authors concluded that "taken together, this pure herbal compound (Withanolide D) may consider as a potential alternative tool with additive effects in conjunction with traditional chemotherapeutic treatment, thereby accelerate the process of conventional drug development".

Oza and coworkers[104] isolated L-asparaginase from the fruits of Withania somnifera. This compound was found to exert a cytotoxic effect on primary leukemia cells obtained from patients newly diagnosed with leukemia (24 h LD_{50} = 1.45 IU/ml).

Yang and coworkers[105] demonstrated the combination of Withaferin A and x-rays as an effective strategy to enhance ionizing radiation (IR)-induced apoptosis in human lymphoma U937 cells. Treatment of U937 cells with Withaferin A (0.5 μM) and IR (10 Gy) induced cell death, whereas treatment with Withaferin A alone did not show a cytotoxic effect. The combined treatment induced apoptosis, increased sub-G1 cell population, increased PARP cleavage, increased ROS, downregulated Bcl-2 and increased p38 and JNK activity. The authors concluded that "the combined regimen with Withaferin A and radiation may offer a better therapeutic strategy to enhance radio sensitivity of tumor cells".

Okamoto and coworkers[106] found that Withaferin A treatment of human myeloid and lymphoid cells suppressed cell growth, induced cell cycle arrest at the G2/M phase, induced partial apoptosis, upregulated heme oxygenase-1 and enhanced autophagy. The authors observed that Withaferin A "has a unique growth suppressive effect on leukemia cells and may serve as a novel therapeutic approach to the treatment of hematological malignancies".

Mckenna and coworkers[107] examined the anticancer activity of Withaferin A in B-cell lymphoma. Treatment of multiple types of human and murine lymphoma cell lines with Withaferin A inhibited cell growth. In several cases, Withaferin A was found to induce cell cycle arrest at the G2/M checkpoint, induce apoptosis, inhibit NF-κB nuclear translocation, decrease protein levels involved in B cell receptor signaling and cell cycle regulation, and inhibit the activity of Hsp90. In vivo studies using synergistic-graft lymphoma cells showed that Withaferin A inhibited the growth of tumor cells without affecting the proliferation of colon epithelial cells. The authors proposed that "the anticancer effects of WA in lymphomas are likely due to its ability to inhibit Hsp90 function and subsequent reduction of critical kinases and cell cycle regulators that are clients of Hsp90".

10.13 – Oral Cancer

Oral cancer begins in the mouth (oral cavity) or in the throat at the back of the mouth (oropharynx). It can develop in the tongue, lips, gums, hard palate, soft palate and other areas. Treatments include surgery, chemotherapy and radiation therapy. A few studies have been conducted to test the effect of Withania somnifera on oral cancer and the results are summarized below.

Panjamurthy and coworkers[108] studied the effect of Withaferin A (WA) on 7,12-dimethylbenz(a)anthracene (DMBA)-induced oral cancer in male golden Syrian hamsters (8-10 weeks old). Animals painted on their left buccal pouches with 5% DMBA in liquid paraffin thrice a week for 14 weeks showed 100% tumor incidence, severe hyperkeratosis, hyperplasia and dysplasia, as well as significantly altered expression of p53 and Bcl-2 proteins. The control group (animals painted with liquid paraffin only) showed none of these changes. Animals treated with WA (20 mg/kg/day, P.O.) for 1 week followed by exposure to DMBA and treatment with WA thrice a week on alternate days for 14 weeks showed no tumor incidence, mild hyperkeratosis, hyperplasia and dysplasia, and significantly less alteration in the expression of p53 and Bcl-2 proteins. In a similar investigation[109], biochemical examination of plasma, erythrocytes and liver samples from hamsters with DMBA-induced oral cancer showed an increase in LPO, cytochrome P450 and cytochrome b5, and a decrease in the levels of GSH, vitamin C, vitamin E, SOD, CAT, GPx and GST compared to controls. Treatment of hamsters with Withaferin A and DMBA showed reversal of the changes induced by DMBA. The authors concluded that "the protective effect of Withaferin A is probably due to its anti-lipid peroxidative and antioxidant functions as well as modulating effect on carcinogen detoxication during DMBA-induced oral carcinogene-sis". Another study[110] demonstrated the circadian time-dependent chemopreventive efficacy of Withaferin A on lipid peroxidation and antioxidants in DMBA-induced oral carcinogenesis in male golden Syrian hamsters.

Yang and coworkers[111] examined the anticancer effect of Withaferin A (WA) against human oral cancer. Treatment of the cancer cell lines HSC-3 and HSC-4 with WA inhibited cell viability and induced apoptosis. WA treatment increased Bim expression in HSC-3 cells and Bax expression in HSC-4 cells, suggesting that WA-induced apoptosis might be associated with cell-specific regula-tion of Bcl-2 family proteins. The authors suggested that "WA may be a potential chemotherapeutic drug candidate against human oral cancer".

Chang and coworkers[112] reported that Withaferin A selectively kills oral cancer cells by regulating oxidative stress-mediated apoptosis. Treating the oral cancer cells Ca9-22 and CAL 27 with Withaferin A reduced cell viability, whereas treating normal HGF-1 cells with Withaferin A showed no effect. Treating Ca9-22 cells with With-aferin A induced G2/M cell cycle arrest, increased annexin V posi-tive expression, increased apoptosis signaling proteins, induced ROS generation, caused mitochondrial membrane depolarization and induced γH2AX-based DNA damage.

10.14 – Kidney Cancer

Kidney cancer arises from kidney tissues. The most common kid-ney cancer is renal carcinoma, which forms in the lining of very small tubules in the kidney. Treatment options include surgery, ablation therapies, biological therapy, embolization and radiother-apy. A few investigations have examined the effect of Withania som-nifera on kidney cancer and some results are summarized below.

Yang and coworkers[113] examined the effect of Withaferin A (WA) on radiation-induced apoptosis in human renal cancer cells (Caki). Treatment of Caki cells with WA+radiation inhibited cell growth, induced apoptosis, increased sub-G1 cell population, induced ROS generation, downregulated Bcl-2, inhibited Akt phosphorylation, and induced PARP cleavage and caspase-3 activity. Although WA and radiation alone were effective, the combination was significantly more effective. The authors concluded that "our study shows that Withaferin A may be used as an effective radiosenisitizer in cancer therapy".

Um and coworkers[114] demonstrated that Withaferin A (WA)-induced apoptosis in Caki cells involves downregulation of the STAT3 pathway. STAT3, a member of the STAT family, is activated in most solid tumors. Treatment of Caki Cells with WA inhibited phosphorylation of STAT3 specifically at Tyr 705, inhibited translocation of STAT3 to the nucleus and suppressed the constitutive activation of JAK2. It was suggested that WA inhibited STAT3 phosphorylation by suppressing JAK2 activation. Treatment of Caki Cells with WA resulted in an increased accumulation of sub-G1 phase cells, PARP cleavage and decreased levels of antiapoptotic Bcl-2, Bcl-xL, survivin and cyclin D1. The authors concluded that "this study demonstrated that Withaferin A induced apoptosis via down-regulation of the STAT3 signaling pathway. Because Withaferin A causes apoptosis, it may be a candidate for a cancer chemopreventative or chemotherapeutic agent".

Choi and coworkers[115] found that Withaferin A treatment of Caki cells induced endoplasmic reticulum (ER) stress and caused upregulation of CHOP. Treatment of Caki cells with N-acetyl cysteine before Withaferin A inhibited ER stress and cell death. The authors concluded that "Taken together, the present study provides strong evidence supporting an important role of the ER stress response in mediating Withaferin A-induced apoptosis".

10.15 – Osteosarcoma

Osteosarcoma is a type of cancer that begins in bone cells. It generally occurs in the long bones that make up the arms and legs, but it can occur in any bone. It mostly affects children, adolescents and young adults. Each year, about 800-900 new cases of osteosarcoma are diagnosed in the United States. Treatment includes surgery, chemotherapy and radiation therapy[116,117]. A few in vitro studies have demonstrated the anticancer activity of Withaferin A in osteosarcoma cell lines and the results are summarized below.

Chen and coworkers[118] found that Withaferin A treatment of the osteosarcoma cell lines U2OS and MG-63 inhibited cell proliferation, induced cell cycle arrest at the G2/M phase, induced transcriptional inactivation of Notch-1 signaling and downregulated MMP-2 and MMP-9 mRNA and protein levels. The authors concluded that "our data provide the first evidence that the down regulation of Notch-1 by Withaferin A may be an effective approach for the treatment of osteosarcoma".

LV and Wang[119] investigated anticancer potential of Withaferin A (WA) in the osteosarcoma cell lines MG-63 and U2OS. Withaferin A treatment of MG-63 and U2OS cells inhibited cell proliferation, induced cell cycle arrest at the G2/M phase, and decreased the levels of cyclin A, cyclin B1, Cdk2 and p-Cdc2 (Tyr15). The authors concluded that "These observations indicate that WA may be used in human osteosarcoma therapy following further clinical investigation".

Li and coworkers[120] evaluated the anticancer potential of Withaferin A in a number of osteosarcoma cell lines: HOS, Saos-2, 143B, MG-63, MNNG, U2OS and Vero. Withaferin A (0.01-10 µM) treatment of these cells inhibited cell proliferation in a dose-dependent manner. IC_{50} values ranged from 0.36 µM (MG-63) to 7.6 µM (Vero). IC_{50} values for doxorubicin ranged from 4.2 µM (MG-63) to 6.3 µM (MNNG). Withaferin A treatment of U2OS cells induced apoptosis, caused ROS generation, caused loss of mitochondrial membrane potential, and induced caspase-3, cytosolic cyt-c and PARP protein expression. The authors concluded that Withaferin A "is a potential candidate for treating osteosarcoma".

References

1   Cancer, World Health Organization, 12 September 2018.
     https://www.who.int/health-topics/cancer
2   Latest global cancer data, World Health Organization, Press Release N 263, 12 September 2018.
3   Cancer types by site. National Cancer Institute, SEER Training Module.
     https://training.seer.cancer.gov/disease/categories/site.html
4   Breast cancer statistics. WCRF International.
     https://www.wcrf.org/dietandcancer/cancer-trends/breast-cancer-statistics
5   What is breast cancer? Centers for Disease Control and Prevention.
     https://www.cdc.gov/cancer/breast/basic_info/what-is-breast-cancer.htm
6   Zhixian Liu, Mengyuan Li, Zehang Jiang and Xiaosheng Wang. A comprehensive immunologic portrait of triple-negative breast cancer. Translational Oncology (2018) 2: 311-329.
7   Bolleddula Jayaprakasam, Yanjun Zhang, Navindra P. Seeram, Muraleedharan G. Nair. Growth inhibition of human tumor cell lines by withanolides from Withania somnifera leaves. Life Sciences (2003) 74: 125-132.
8   Gottumukkala V. Subbaraju, Mulabagal Vanisree, Chirravuri V. Rao, Chillara Sivaramakrishna, Pratha Sridhar, Bolleddula Jayaprakasam, and Muraleedharam G Nair. Ashwagandhanolide, a bioactive dimeric thiowithanolide isolated from the roots of Withania somnifera. J. Nat. Prod (2006) 69: 1790 – 1792.
9   Vanisree Mulabagal, Gottumukkala V. Subbaraju, Chirravuri V. Rao, Chillara Sivaramakrishna, David L. Dewitt, Daniel Holmes, Bokyung Sung, Bharat B. Aggarwal, Hsin-Sheng Tsay and Muraleedharan G. Nair. Withanolide Sulfoxide from Aswagandha roots inhibits nuclear transcription factor-kappa-B, cyclooxygenase and tumor cell proliferation. Phytother Res (2009) 23 (7): 987-92.
10   Rajeev Nema, Sarita Khare, Parul Jain and Alka pradhan. Anticancer activity of Withania somnifera (leaves) flavonoids compound. Int. J. Pharm. Sci. Rev.

Res (2013) 19(1) n 21, 103-106.

11 Mary Kaileh, Wim Vanden Berghe, Elke Boone, Tamer Essawi, Guy Haegeman. Screening of indigenous Palestinian medicinal plants for potential anti-inflammatory and cytotoxic activity. Journal of Ethnopharmacology (2007) 113 (3): 510-516.

12 Silvia D. Stan, Eun-Ryeong Hahm, Renaud Warin, and Shivendra V. Singh. Withaferin A causes FOXO3a and Bim-dependent apoptosis and inhibits growth of human breast cancer cells in vivo. Cancer Res (2008) 68 (18):7661-7669.

13 Silvia D. Stan, Yan Zeng, and Shivendra V. Singh. Ayurvedic medicine constituent Withaferin A causes G2 and M phase cell cycle arrest in human breast cancer cells. Nutr Cancer (2008) 60 (suppl 1) 51-60.

14 Joomin Lee, Eun-Ryeong Hahm and Shivendra V. singh. Withaferin A inhibits activation of signal transducer and activator of transcription 3 in human breast cancer cells. Carcinogenesis (2010) 31 (11): 1991-1998.

15 Eun-Ryeong Hahm, Joomin Lee, Yi Huang, and Shivendra V. Singh. Withaferin A suppresses estrogen receptor-α expression in human breast cancer cells. Mol Carcinog (2011) 50 (8): 614-624.

16 Eun-Ryeong Hahm, Joomin Lee, and Shivendra V. Singh. Role of mitogen-activated protein kinases and Mcl-1 in apoptosis induction by Withaferin A in human breast cancer cells. Mol Carcinog (2014) 53 (11): 907-916.

17 Eun-Ryeong Hahm, Michelle B. Moura, Eric E. Kelly, Bennett Van Houten, Sruti Shiva, Shivendra V. Singh. Withaferin A-induced apoptosis in human breast cancer cells is mediated by reactive oxygen species. PLOS ONE (2011) 6 (8); 1-12 e23354.

18 Eun-Ryeong Hahm and Shivendra V. Singh. Autophagy fails to alter Withaferin A-mediated lethality in human breast cancer cells. Curr Cancer Drug Targets (2013) 13(6): 640-650.

19 Eun-Ryeong Hahm, Shivendra V. Singh. Withaferin A-induced apoptosis in human breast cancer cells is associated with suppression of inhibitor of apoptosis family protein expression. Cancer Letters (2013) 334: 101-108.

20 Jose T. Thaiparambil, Laura Bender, Thota Ganesh, Erik Kline, Pritty Patel, Yuan Liu, Mourad Tighiouart, Paula M. Vertino, R. Donald Harvey, Anapatricia Garcia and Adam I. Marcus. Withaferin A inhibits breast cancer invasion and metastasis at sub-cytotoxic doses by inducing vimentin disassembly and serine 56 phosphorylation. Int. J. Cancer (2011) 129: 2744-2755.

21 Zhen Yang, Anapatricia Garcia, Songli Xu, Doris R. Powell, Paula M. Vertino, Shivendra Singh, Adam I. Marcus. Withania somnifera root extract inhibits mammary cancer metastasis and epithelial to mesenchymal transition. PLOS ONE (2013) 8 (9): 1-12 e75069.

22 Maliyakkal N, Udupa N, Pai KSR, Rangarajan A. Cytotoxic and apoptotic activities of extracts of Withania somnifera and Tinospora cordifolia in human breast cancer cells. International Journal of Applied Research in Natural products (2013) 6 (4):1-10.

23 Xuan Zhang, Ridhwi Mukerji, Abbas K Samadi and Mark S Cohen. Down-regulation of estrogen receptor-alpha and rearranged during transfection tyrosine kinase is associated with Withaferin A-induced apoptosis in MCF-7 breast cancer cells. BMC Complementary and Alternative Medicine (2011) 11: 84.

24 Kamel F. Khazal, Temesgen Samuel, Donald L. Hill, and Clinton J. Grubbs. Effect of an extract of Withania somnifera root on estrogen receptor-positive mammary carcinomas. Anticancer Res (2013) 33(4): 1519-1523.

25 Kamel F. Khazal, Donald L. Hill and Clinton J. Grubbs. Effect of Withania

somnifera root extract on spontaneous estrogen receptor-negative mammary cancer in MMTV/ Neu mice. Anticancer Res (2014) 34 (11): 6327-6332.

26 Kamel F. Khazal, Donald L. Hill. Withania somnifera extract reduces the invasiveness of MDA-MB-231 breast cancer and inhibits cytokines associated with metastasis. Journal of Cancer Metastasis and Treatment (2015) 1 (2): 94-100.

27 Eun-Ryeong Hahm, Joomin Lee, Su-Hyeong Kim, Anuradha Sehrawat, Julie A. Arlotti, Sruti S. Shiva, Rohit Bhargava, Shivendra V. Singh. Metabolic alterations in mammary cancer prevention by Withaferin A in a clinically relevant model. J Natl Cancer Inst (2013) 105: 1111-1122.

28 Su-Hyeong Kim and Shivendra V. Singh. Mammary cancer chemoprevention by Withaferin A is accompanied by in vivo suppression of self-renewal of cancer stem cells. Cancer Prev Res (2014) 7 (7): 738-747.

29 Marie L. Antony, Joomin Lee, Eun-Ryeong Hahm, Su-Hyeong Kim, Adam I. Marcus, Vandana Kumari, Xinhua Ji, Zhen Yang, Courtney L. Vowell, Peter Wipf, Guy T. Uechi, Nathan A. Yates, Guillermo Romero, Saumendra N. Sarkar, and Shivendra V. Singh. Growth arrest by the antitumor steroidal lactone Withaferin A in human breast cancer cells is associated with down-regulation and covalent binding at cysteine 303 of β-tubulin. Journal of Biological Chemistry (2014) 289 (3): 1852-1865.

30 Arumugam Nagalingam, Panjamurthy Kuppusamy, Shivendra Singh, Dipali Sharma and Neeraj K. Saxena. Mechanistic elucidation of the antitumor properties of Withaferin A in breast cancer. Cancer Res (2014) 74 (9): 2617-2629.

31 Joomin Lee, Eun-Ryeong Hahm, Adam I. Marcus, and Shivendra V. Singh. Withaferin A inhibits experimental epithelial-mesenchymal transition in MCF-10A cells and suppresses vimentin protein level in vivo in breast tumors. Mol Carcinog (2015) 54 (6): 417-429.

32 N. Muninathan, P. Mohanalakshmi, Ambareesha Kondam K, S. Malliga. Effect of paclitaxel along with Withania somnifera on lactate dehydrogenase enzyme activity changes in 7,12 dimethylbenz(a) anthracene induced breast cancer Wistar rats. National Journal of Medical Research and Yoga Science (2015) 1 (2): 25-27.

33 Colorectal cancer statistics, World Cancer Research Fund. https://www.wcrf.org/dietandcancer/cancer-trends/colorectal-cancer-statistics

34 Amreen A. Siddique, Pallavi Joshi, Laxminarain Misra, Neelam S. Sangwan, Mahendra P. Darokar. 5,6-de-epoxy-5-en-7-one-17-hydroxy Withaferin A, a new cytotoxic steroid from Withania somnifera L. Dunal leaves. Nat Prod Res (2014) 28 (6): 392-8.

35 Srinivas Koduru, Raj Kumar, Sowmyalakshmi Srinivasan, Mark B. Evers, and Chendil Damodaran. Notch-1 inhibition by Withaferin A: A therapeutic target against colon carcinogenesis. Mol Cancer Ther (2010) 9 (1): 202- 210.

36 Suman Suman, Trinath P. Das, Suman Sirimulla, Houda Alatassi, Murali K. Ankem, Chendil Damodaran. Withaferin – A suppress AKT induced tumor growth in colorectal cancer cells. Oncotarget (2016) 7(12): 13854 – 13864.

37 Tania Das, Kumar Singha Roy, Tulika Chakrabarti, Sibabrata Mukhopadhyay, Susanta Roychoudhury. Withaferin A modulates the spindle assembly checkpoint by degradation of Mad2–Cdc20 complex in colorectal cancer cell lines. Biochemical Pharmacology (2014) 91: 31–39.

38 Bu Young Choi, and Bong-Woo Kim. Withaferin – A inhibits colon cancer cell growth by blocking STAT3 transcriptional activity. Journal Of Cancer Prevention (2015) 20: 185-92.

39 Govindan Muralikrishnan, Amit K Dinda & Faiyaz Shakeel. Immunomodulatory effects of Withania somnifera on azoxymethane induced

experimental colon cancer in mice. Immunological Investigations (2010) 39 (7): 688-98.

40 Govindan Muralikrishnan, Safiullah Amanullah, Mohamed I Basha, Amit K Dinda & Faiyaz Shakeel. Modulating effect of Withania somnifera on TCA cycle enzymes and electron transport chain in azoxymethane induced colon cancer in mice. Immunopharmacology and Immunotoxicology (2010) 32 (3): 523-7.

41 L. Dusek, J. Muzik, D. Maluskova, L, Snajdrova. Epidemiology of cervical cancer: international comparison. Cervical Cancer Screening Program in the Czech Republic. https://www.cervix.cz/index-en.php?pg=professionals–cervical-cancer-epidemiology–international-comparison

42 Cervical Cancer Overview, National Cervical Cancer Coalition. https://www.nccc-online.org/hpvcervical-cancer/cervical-cancer-overview/

43 Radha Munagala, Hina Kausar, Charu Munjal and Ramesh C. Gupta. Withaferin A induces p53-dependent apoptosis by repression of HPV oncogenes and upregulation of tumor suppressor proteins in human cervical cancer cells. Carcinogenesis (2011) 32(11); 1697-2011.

44 Zheng-Guo Cui, Jin-Lan Piao, Mati U. R. Rehman, Ryohei Ogawa, Peng Li, Qing-Li Zhao, Takashi Kondo, Hidekuni Inadera. Molecular mechanisms of hyperthermia-induced apoptosis enhanced by Withaferin A. European Journal of Pharmacology (2014) 723: 99 – 107.

45 Daehyung Lee, In-Hye Lim, Eon-Gi Sung, Joo-Young Kim, In-Hwan Song, Yoon Ki Park and Tae- Jin Lee. Withaferin A inhibits matrix metalloproteinase-9 activity by suppressing the Akt signaling pathway. Oncology Reports (2013) 30: 933- 948.

46 Dong Eun Kim. Withaferin A inhibits PMA-induced MMP-9 expression in human cervical carcinoma Caski cells. Journal of Life Science (2013) 23(3): 355-360.

47 Abhimanyu Kumar Jha, Mohsen Nikbakht, Neena Capalash and Jagdeep Kaur. Demethylation of RARβ2 gene promoter by Withania somnifera in HeLa cell line. European Journal of Medicinal Plants (2014) 4(5): 503-510.

48 Li Ye and Qian Song. Withaferin A suppresses anti-apoptotic BCL2, Bcl-xL, XIAP and survivin genes in cervical carcinoma cells. Tropical Journal of Pharmaceutical Research (2015) 14 (12): 2201-2206.

49 Satish Kumar, Lingaraja Jena, Maheswata Sahoo, Tapaswini Nayak, Kanchan Mohod, Sangeeta Daf, and Ashok K. Varma. The in silico approach to identify a unique plant-derived inhibitor against E6 and E7 oncogenic proteins of high-risk human papillomavirus 16 and 18. Avicenna J Med Biochem (2016) June; 4(1): e33958.

50 Prostate cancer statistics. World Cancer Research Fund. https://www.wcrf.org/dietandcancer/cancer-trends/prostate-cancer-statistics

51 Sowmylakshmi Srinivasan, Rama S. Ranga, Ravshan Burikhanov, Seong-Su Han, and Damodaran Chendil. Par-4-dependent apoptosis by the dietary compound Withaferin A in prostate cancer cells. Cancer Res (2007) 67(1): 246-253.

52 Ram V. Roy, Suman Suman, Tripathi P. Das, Joe E. Luevano, and Chendil Damodaran. Withaferin A, a steroidal lactone from Withania somnifera, induces mitotic catastrophe and growth arrest in prostate cancer cells. Journal of Natural Products (2013) 76:1909-1915.

53 Yukihiro Nishikawa, Daisuke Okuzaki, Kohshiro Fukushima, Satomi Mukai, Shouichi Ohno, Yuki Ozaki, Norikazu Yabuta, Hiroshi Nojima. Withaferin A induces cell death selectively in androgen-independent prostate cancer cells but not in normal fibroblast cells. PLOS ONE. doi: 10.1371/journal.pone.0134137

54 K. V. K. Rao, Stanley A. Schwartz, Hari Krishnan Nair, Ravikumar
    Aalinkeel, Supriya Mahajan, Ram Chawda and Madhavan P. N. Nair. Plant
    derived products as a source of cellular growth inhibitory phytochemicals on
    PC-3M, DU-145 and LNCaP prostate cell lines. Current Science (2004) 87
    (11): 1585-1588.

55 Ravikumar Aalinkeel, Zihua Hu, Bindukumar B. Nair, Donald E. Sykes,
    Jessica L. Reynolds, Supriya D. Mahajan and Stanley A. Schwartz. Genomic
    analysis highlights the role of the JAK-STAT signaling in the anti-proliferative
    effects of dietary flavonoid- Ashwagandha in prostate cancer cells. eCAM
    2010:7 (2) 177-178.

56 Bhuwaneshor Yadav, Amarjeet Bajaj, Mridula Saxena, Anil Kumar Saxena.
    In vitro anticancer activity of the root, stem and leaves of Withania somnifera
    against various human cancer lines. Indian J Pharm Sci (2010) 72(5): 659-
    663.

57 Shailesh Singh, Rajesh Singh, James Lillard jr, and William Grizzle.
    Inhibition of prostate tumor growth by potentiating antitumor immune
    response using natural product (162.46) The Journal of Immunology (2012)
    188 (1 suppl) 162.46.

58 Lung cancer statistics. World Research Fund. American Institute for Cancer
    Research. https://www.wcrf.org/dietandcancer/cancer-trends/lung-cancer-
    statistics

59 M. Iqbal Choudhary, Shabir Hussain, Sammar Yousuf, Ahsana Dar,
    Mudassar, Atta-ur-Rahman. Chlorinated and diepoxy withanolides from
    Withania somnifera and their cytotoxic effects against human lung cancer cell
    line. Phytochemistry (2010) 71 (17-18): 2205-2209.

60 N, Singh, S. P. Singh, R. Nath, D. R. Singh, M. L. Gupta, R. P. Kohli and K.
    P. Bhargava. Prevention of urethane-induced lung adenomas by Withania
    somnifera (L.) Dunal in albino mice. International Journal of Crude Drug
    Research (1986) 24 (2): 90-100.

61 Rajeev Nema, Sarita Khare, Parul Jain and Alka Pradhan. Anticancer activity
    of Withania somnifera (leaves) flavonoids compound. Int. J. Pharm. Sci. Rev.
    Res (2013) 19 (1); n21, 103-106.

62 Palaniyandi Senthilnathan, Radhakrishnan Padmavathi, Venkataraman
    Magesh and Dhanapal Sakthisekaran. Chemotherapeutic efficacy of paclitaxel
    in combination with Withania somnifera on benzo(a)pyrene-induced
    experimental lung cancer. Cancer Sci (2006) 97 (7):658-664.

63 Palaniyandi Senthilnathan, Radhakrishnan Padmavathi, Venkatraman
    Magesh and Dhanapal Sakthisekaran. Stabilization of membrane bound
    enzyme profiles and lipid peroxidation by Withania somnifera along with
    paclitaxel on benzo(a)pyrene induced experimental lung cancer. Molecular
    and Cellular Biochemistry (2006) 292: 13-17.

64 Palaniyandi Senthilnathan, Radhakrishan Padmavathi, Venkataraman Magesh
    and Dhanapal Sakthisekaran. Modulation of TCA enzymes and electron
    transport chain systems in experimental lung cancer. Life Sciences (2006) 78
    (9): 1010-1014.

65 Yong Cai, Zhao-ying Sheng, Yun Chen. Chong Bai, Effect of Withaferin A
    on A549 cellular proliferation and apoptosis in non small cell lung cancer.
    Asia Pacific Journal of Cancer Prevention (2014) 15: 1711-1714.

66 Xi Liu, Lei Chen, Tao Liang, Xiao-dong Tian, Yang Liu, Tao Zhang.
    Withaferin A induces mitochondrial-dependent apoptosis in non-small cell
    lung cancer cells via generation of reactive oxygen species. JBUON (2017) 22
    (1): 244-250.

67 Jai Prakash, S. K. Gupta, V. Kochupillai, N. Singh, Y. K. Gupta and S. Joshi.
    Chemopreventive activity of Withania somnifera in experimentally induced

fibrosarcoma tumours in Swiss albino mice. Phytother. Res (2001) 15: 240 – 244.

68 Davis L, Kuttan G. Effect of Withania somnifera on 20–methylcholanthrene induced fibrosarcoma. J Exp Clin Cancer Res (2000) 19 (2): 165-167.

69 Kaileh M, Vanden Berghe W, Boone E, Essawi T, Haegeman G. Screening of indigenous Palestanian medicinal plants for potential anti-inflammatory and cytotoxic activity. J Ethnopharmacol (2007) 113 (3): 510-6.

70 Nashi Widodo, Kamalajit Kaur, Bhupal G. Shrestha, Yasuomi Takagi, Tetsuro Ishii, Renu Wadhwa, and Sunil C. Kaul. Selective killing of cancer cells by leaf extract of Ashwagandha: identification of a tumor-inhibitory factor and the first molecular insights to its effect. Clin Cancer Res (2007) 13 (7): 2298-2306.

71 Nashi Widodo, Yasuomi Takagi, Bhupal G. Shrestha, Tetsuro Ishii, Sunil C. Kaul, Renu Wadhwa. Selective killing of cancer cells by leaf extract of Ashwagandha: components, activity and pathway analyses. Cancer Letters (2008) 262: 37-47.

72 Key Statistics about Neuroblastoma, American Cancer Society. https://www.cancer.org/cancer/neuroblastoma/about/key-statistics.html

73 Hardeep Kataria, Renu Wadhwa, Sunil C. Kaul, Gurucharan Kaur. Withania somnifera water extract as a potential candidate for differentiation based therapy of human neuroblastomas. PLOS ONE (2013) 8 (1) e55316.

74 Lisette P. Yco, Gabor Mocz, John Opoku-Ansah and Andre S. Bachmann. Withaferin A inhibits STAT3 and induces tumor cell death in neuroblastomas and multiple myeloma. Biochemistry Insights (2014) 7: 1-13.

75 Skin Cancers, World Health Organization. https://www.who.int/uv/faq/skincancer/en/index1.html

76 Leemol Davis, Girija Kuttan. Effect of Withania somnifera on DMBA induced carcinogenesis. Journal of Ethnopharmacology (2001) 75: 165-168.

77 Jai Prakash, Suresh Kumar Gupta, Amit Kumar Dinda. Withania somnifera root extract prevents DMBA induced squamous cell carcinoma of skin in Swiss albino mice. Nutrition and Cancer (2002) 42(1): 91-7.

78 Bandhuvula Padmavathi, Pramod C. Rath, Araga Ramesha Rao and Rana Pratap Singh. Roots of Withania somnifera inhibit forestomach and skin carcinogenesis in mice. eCAM 2005: 2 (1) 99-105.

79 P. V. Leyon and G. Kuttan. Effect of Withania somnifera on B16F-10 melanoma induced metastasis in mice. Phytother. Res (2004) 18: 118-122.

80 S. Mathur, P. Kaur, M. Sharma, A. Katyal, B. Singh, M. Tiwari, R. Chandra. The treatment of skin carcinoma, induced by UV B radiation, using 1-oxo-5β,6β-epoxy-witha-2-enolide, isolated from the roots of Withania somnifera, in a rat model. Phytomedicine (2004) 11:452-460.

81 Eleonore Mayola, Cindy Gallerne, Davide Degli Esposti, Cecile Martel, Shazib Pervaiz, Lionel Larue, Brigitte Debuire, Antoinette Lemoine, Catherine Brenner, Christophe Lemaire. Withaferin A induces apoptosis in human melanoma cells through generation of reactive oxygen species and down-regulation of Bcl-2. Apoptosis (2011) 16: 1014-1027.

82 Babli Halder, Shruti Singh, Suman S. Thakur. Withania somnifera root extract has potent cytotoxic effect against human malignant melanoma cells. PLOS ONE 10 (9) e0137498. doi: 10.1371/journal.pone.0137498.

83 P. Uma Devi, Ravindra Kamath and B S Satish Rao. Radiosensitization of a mouse melanoma by Withaferin A: in vivo studies. Indian Journal of Experimental Biology (2000) 38: 432-437.

84 Pathirissery Uma Devi and Ravindra Kamath. Radiosensitizing effect of Withaferin A combined with hyperthermia on mouse fibrosarcoma and melanoma. J. Radiat. Res (2003) 44: 1-6.

85 Guruprasad Kalthur and Uma Devi Pathirissery. Enhancement of the
    response of B 16F1 melanoma to fractionated radiotherapy and prolongation
    of survival by Withaferin A and/or hyperthermia. Integrative Cancer
    Therapies (2010) 9 (4): 370-377.
86 Guruprasad Kalthur, Srinivasa Mutalik, Uma Devi Pathirissery. Effect of
    Withaferin A on the development and decay of thermotolerance in B16F1
    melanoma: a preliminary study. Integrative Cancer Therapies (2009) 8(1): 93-
    97.
87 Wenjuan Li and Yunfeng Zhao. Withaferin A suppresses tumor promoter
    12-O-tetradecanoylphorbol 13-acetate-induced decreases in isocitrate
    dehydrogenase 1 activity and mitochondrial function in skin epidermal JB6
    cells. Cancer Science (2013) 104 (2): 143-148.
88 Li W, Zhang C, Du H, Huang V, Sun B, Harris JP, Richardson Q, Shen X,
    Jin R, Li G, Kevil CG, Gu X, Shi R, Zhao Y. Withaferin A suppresses the up-
    regulation of acetyl-coA carboxylase 1 and skin tumor formation in a skin
    carcinogenesis mouse model. Mol Carcinog (2016) 55 (11): 1739-1746.
89 Types & stages of ovarian cancer. National Ovarian Cancer Coalition.
    http://ovarian.org/about-ovarian-cancer/what-is-ovarian-cancer/types-a-stages
90 Xuan Zhang, Abbas K. Samadi, Katherine F. Roby, Barbara Timmermann,
    Mark S. Cohen. Inhibition of cell growth and induction of apoptosis in
    ovarian carcinoma cell lines CaOV3 and SKOV3 by natural withanolide
    Withaferin A. Gynecologic Oncology (2012) 124: 606-612.
91 Sham S. Kakar, Venkatakrishna R. Jala, and Miranda Y. Fong. Synergistic
    cytotoxic action of Cisplatin and Withaferin A on ovarian cancer cell lines.
    Biochem Biophys Res Commun (2012) 423 (4): 819-825.
92 Sham S. Kakar, Mariusz Z. Ratajczak, Karen S. Powell, Mana
    Moghadamfalahi, Donald M. Miller, Surinder K. Batra, Sanjay K. Singh.
    Withaferin A alone and in combination with Cisplatin suppresses growth and
    metastasis of ovarian cancer by targeting putative cancer stem cells. PLOS
    ONE (2014) 9 (9): e107596.
93 Miranda Y, Fong, Shunying Jin, Madhavi Rane, Raj K. Singh, Ramesh Gupta,
    Sham S. Kakar. Withaferin A synergizes the therapeutic effect of doxorubicin
    through ROS- mediated autophagy in ovarian cancer. PLOS ONE (2012)
    7(7): e42265.
94 Animesh Barua, Michael J, Bradaric, Pincas Bitterman, Jacques S.
    Abramowicz, Sameer Sharma, Sanjib Basu, Heather Lopez, Janice M. Bahr.
    Dietary supplementation of Ashwagandha (Withania somnifera, Dunal)
    enhances NK cell function in ovarian tumors in the laying hen model of
    spontaneous ovarian cancer. American Journal of Reproductive Immunology
    (2013) 70: 538 – 550.
95 What is pancreatic cancer? Pancreatic Cancer Action Network.
    https://www.pancan.org/facing-pancreatic-cancer/about-pancreatic-cancer/
    what-is-pancreatic-cancer/
96 Yanke Yu, Adel Hamza, Tao Zhang, Mancang Gu, Peng Zou, Bryan
    Newman, Yanyan Li, A. A. Leslie Gunatilaka, Luke Whitesell, Chang-Guo
    Zhan, and Duxin Sun. Withaferin A targets heat shock protein 90 in
    pancreatic cancer cells. Biochem Pharmacol (2010) 79 (4); 542–551.
97 Abhinav Grover, Ashutosh Shandilya, Vibhuti Agrawal, Piyush Pratik, Divya
    Bhasme, Virendra S Bisaria, Durai Sundar. Hsp90/Cdc37 chaperone/ co-
    chaperone complex, a novel junction anticancer target elucidated by the
    mode of action of herbal drug Withaferin A. BMC Bioinformatics (2011) 12
    (suppl 1): S30.
98 Xu Li, Feng Zhu, Jianxin Jiang, Chengyi Sun, Xin Wang, Ming Shen, Rui
    Tian, Chengjian Shi, Meng Xu, Feng Peng, Xingjun Guo, Min Wang, Renyi

Qin. Synergistic antitumor activity of Withaferin A combined with Oxaliplatin triggers reactive oxygen species-mediated inactivation of the P13K/AKT pathway in human pancreatic cancer cells. Cancer Letters (2015) 357: 219–230.

99 Sayantani Sarkar, Chandan Mandal, Rajender Sangwan and Chitra Mandal. Coupling G2/M arrest to the Wnt/β-catenin pathway restrains pancreatic adenocarcinoma. Society for Endocrinology (2014) 21 (1): 113-125.

100 V. Senthil, S. Ramadevi, V. Venkatakrishnan, P. Giridharan, B. S. Lakshmi, R. A. Vishwakarma, A. Balakrishnan. Withanolide induces apoptosis in HL-60 leukemia cells via mitochondria mediated cytochrome C release and caspase activation. Chemico-Biological Interactions (2007) 167: 19-30.

101 Fayaz Malik, Ajay Kumar, Shashi Bhushan, Sheema Khan, Aruna Bhatia, Krishan Avtar Suri, Ghulam Nabi Qazi, Jaswant Singh. Reactive oxygen species generation and mitochondrial dysfunction in the apoptotic cell death of human myeloid leukemia HL-60 cells by a dietary compound Withaferin A with concomitant protection by n-acetyl cysteine. Apoptosis (2007) 12: 2155-2133.

102 Chandan Mandal, Avijit Dutta, Asish Mallick, Sarmila Chandra, Laxminarain Misra, Rajender S. Sangwan, Chitra Mandal. Withaferin A induces apoptosis by activating p38 mitogen-activated protein kinase signaling cascade in leukemic cells of lymphoid and myeloid origin through mitochondrial death cascade. Apoptosis (2008) 13: 1450-1464.

103 Susmita Mondal, Chandan Mandal, Rajender Sangwan, Sarmila Chandra, Chitra Mandal. Withanolide D induces apoptosis in leukemia by targeting the activation of neutral sphingomyelinase-ceramide cascade mediated by synergistic activation of c-Jun N-terminal kinase and p38 mitogen-activated protein kinase. Molecular Cancer (2010) 9:239.

104 Vishal P. Oza, Pritesh P. Parmar, Sushil Kumar, R. B. Subramanian. Anticancer properties of highly purified L-Asparaginase from Withania somnifera L. against acute lymphoblastic leukemia. Appl Biochem Biotechnol (2010) 160: 1833–1840.

105 Eun Sun Yang, Min Jung Choi, Jin Hee Kim, Kyeong Sook Choi, Taeg Kyu Kwon. Combination of Withaferin A and X-ray irradiation enhances apoptosis in U937 cells. Toxicology in Vitro (2011) 25: 1803-1810.

106 Shuichiro Okamoto, Takayuki Tsujioka, Shin-ichiro Suemori, Jun-ichiro Kida, Toshinori Kondo, Yumi Tohyama and Kaoru Tohyama. Withaferin A suppresses the growth of myelodysplasia and leukemia cell lines by inhibiting cell cycle progression. Cancer Science (2016) 107(9): 1302–1314.

107 MK Mckenna, BW Gachuki, SS Alhakeem, KN Oben, VM Rangnekar, RC Gupta and S Bondada. Anti-cancer activity of Withaferin A in B-cell lymphoma. Cancer Biology & Therapy, (2015) 16(7): 1088-1098.

108 Kuppusamy Panjamurthy, Shanmugam Manoharan, Madhavan Ramados Nirmal, Lakshmanan Vellaichamy. Protective role of Withaferin-A on immunoexpression of p53 and bcl-2 in 7,12-dimethylbenz(a)anthracene-induced experimental oral carcinogenesis. Invest New Drugs (2009) 27: 447-452.

109 S Manoharan, K Panjamurthy, Venugopal P Menon, S Balakrishnan & Linsa Mary Alias. Protective effect of Withaferin A in 7,12-dimethylbenz(a)anthracene induced oral carcinogenesis in hamsters. Indian Journal of Experimental Biology (2009) 47: 16-23.

110 Shanmugam Manoharan, Kuppusamy Panjamurthy, Subramanian Balakrishnan, Kalaiarasan Vasudevan, Lakshmanan Vellaichamy. Circadian time-dependent chemopreventive potential of Withaferin A in 7,12-dimethylbenz(a)anthracene induced oral carcinogenesis. Pharmacological

Reports (2009) 61:719-726.

111 In-Hyoung Yang, Lee-Han Kim, Ji-ae-shin, Sung-Dae Cho. Chemotherapeutic effect of Withaferin A in human oral cancer cells. Journal of Cancer Therapy (2015) 6: 735-742.

112 Hsueh-Wei Chang, Ruei-Nian Li, Hui-Ru Wang, Jing-Ru Liu, Jen-Yang Tang, Hurng-Wern Huang, Yu-Hsuan Chan and Ching-Yu Yen. Withaferin A induces oxidative stress-mediated apoptosis and DNA damage in oral cancer cells. Frontiers in Physiology (2017) 8, Article 634. doi: 10.3389/fphys.2017.00634

113 Eun Sun Yang, Min Jung Choi, Jin Hee Kim, Kyeong Sook Choi, Taeg Kyu Kwon. Withaferin A enhances radiation-induced apoptosis in Caki cells through induction of reactive oxygen species, Bcl-2 downregulation and Akt inhibition. Chemico-Biological Interactions (2011) 190: 9-15.

114 Hee Jung Um, Kyoung-jin Min, Dong Eun Kim, Taeg Kyu Kwon. Withaferin A inhibits JAK/STAT3 signaling and induces apoptosis of human renal carcinoma Caki cells. Biochemical and Biophysical Research Communications (2012) 427: 24-29.

115 Min Jung Choi, Eun Jung Park, Kyoung Jin Min, Jong-Wook Park, Taeg Kyu Kwon. Endoplasmic reticulum stress mediates Withaferin A-induced apoptosis in human renal carcinoma cells. Toxicology in Vitro (2011) 25 (3): 692-698.

116 Osteosarcoma, Rare Disease Database. National Organization for Rare Disorders. https://rarediseases.org/rare-diseases/osteosarcoma/

117 Key statistics for osteosarcoma, American Cancer Society. https://www.cancer.org/cancer/osteosarcoma/about/key-statistics.html

118 Yang Chen, Xiang Zhen Han, Wei Wang, Ren Tao Zhao and Xiao Li. Withaferin A inhibits osteosarcoma cells through inactivation of Notch-1 signaling. Bangladesh J Pharmacol (2014) 9: 364-370.

119 Ting-Zhuo LV and Guang-Shun Wang. Antiproliferation potential of Withaferin A on human osteosarcoma cells via the inhibition of G2/M checkpoint proteins. Experimental and Therapeutic Medicine (2015) 10: 323-329.

120 A-X Li, M. Sun, X. Li. Withaferin A induces apoptosis in osteosarcoma U2OS cell line via generation of ROS and disruption of mitochondrial membrane potential. European Review for Medical and Pharmacological Sciences (2017) 21 (6): 1368-1374.

11 – Cardioprotective Activity

11.1 – Introduction

Cardiovascular disease (CVD) is a group of disorders of the heart and blood vessels. It is the leading cause of death globally. An estimated 17.9 million people died from CVDs in 2016[1]. In the United States, an estimated 647,000 people die of heart disease every year. Behavioral risk factors include tobacco use, unhealthy diet and obesity, physical inactivity, substance abuse and excessive consumption of alcohol[2]. Treatment options include lifestyle alterations, medication and surgery. A number of studies have examined the effect of Withania somnifera on cardiovascular diseases and the results are summarized below.

11.2 – Summary of results

Mohanty and coworkers[3] evaluated the cardioprotective effect of a hydro-alcoholic extract of Withania somnifera root (WS) on isoproterenol (ISP)-induced myocardial necrosis in rats. Wistar male albino rats treated with saline for 4 weeks and injected with ISP (85 mg/kg, S.C.) on days 29 and 30 showed the following changes compared to controls:

- increased LPO, decreased glutathione content and decreased activities of antioxidant enzymes in heart tissue
- decreased activities of LDH and CPK myocardial enzymes
- left ventricular dysfunction

Rats treated with WS (25-100 mg/kg/day, P.O.) for 4 weeks and injected with ISP (85 mg/kg, S.C.) on days 29 and 30 showed decreased myocardial LPO, enhanced antioxidant status, increased myocardial LDH and CPK, and improved ventricular function. Histopathological studies of myocardial tissue in the ISP-only group showed myocardial damage. Pretreatment with WS (50 or 100 mg/kg) prevented ISP-induced myonecrosis. The authors concluded that "clinical trials should be conducted to support [WS] therapeutic use in ischaemic heart diseases".

Khalil and coworkers[4] demonstrated the cardioprotective effect of an ethanol (70%) extract of Withania somnifera leaf (WSLEt) on isoproterenol (ISP)-induced myocardial infarction (MI) in rats. Adult male Wistar albino rats treated with distilled water for 4 weeks and injected with ISO (85 mg/kg, S.C.) on days 29 and 30 showed the following changes compared to controls:

- increased heart weight
- increased serum cardiac troponin I (cTnI), TC, TG, VLDL-C and decreased HDL-C
- increased LPO and decreased SOD, GPx, GRx and GST in heart tissue

Rats treated with WSLEt (100 mg/kg/day, S.C.) for 4 weeks followed by injection with ISO (85 mg/kg, S.C.) on days 29 and 30 showed a reversal of these changes.

Histopathological examination of heart tissues in the ISO group showed cardiac muscle fibers with muscle separation, edematous intramuscular space and inflammatory cells. The morphology in the WSLEt+IPO group was similar to normal tissue. The authors concluded that "W. somnifera leaves have the potential to be used as cardioprotective agents by protecting cardiac tissue against oxidative damage".

Hamza and coworkers[5] investigated the effect of a standard extract of Withania somnifera roots and leaves (WIT) on doxorubicin (DXR)-induced cardiac toxicity. Adult male albino Wistar rats treated with distilled water (5 ml/kg/day, P.O.) for 14 days and injected with a single dose of DXR (10 mg/kg, i.p.), showed the following changes after 7 days compared to controls:

- increased serum AST
- increased LPO, protein carbonyl, CAT, MPO and heart-specific calcium content in heart tissue
- decreased SOD and total antioxidant capacity in heart tissue
- increased TUNEL-positive cells and Bcl-2 expression in heart tissue
- myocardial histopathological lesions

Rats treated with WIT (300 mg/kg/day, P.O.) for 14 days and injected with DXR (10 mg/kg, i.p.) 7 days after the commencement of WIT treatment showed a reversal of these changes. The authors concluded that "The protective effect of WIT may be mediated through its antioxidant, anti-inflammatory and calcium antagonistic properties".

Gupta and coworkers[6] evaluated the efficacy of a hydro-alcoholic lyophilized extract of Withania somnifera (WS) to mitigate myocardial injury induced by ischemia and reperfusion in rats. Wistar albino rats treated with saline for 30 days and subjected to occlusion of the left anterior descending (LAD) coronary artery for 45 minutes, followed by reperfusion for 60 minutes showed the following changes compared to controls:

- decreased mean arterial pressure, depressed heart rate, decreased left ventricular peak (+)LVdP/dt and (−)LVdP/dt

- increased LPO and decreased GSH, SOD, CAT, LDH and CPK in heart tissue

Rats treated with WS (50 mg/kg/day, P.O.) for 30 days and subjected to the same ischemia and reperfusion showed attenuation of most of these changes. Histopathological studies of myocardial tissues of rats treated with saline and subjected to ischemia and reperfusion showed myonecrosis, edema and infiltration of inflammatory cells compared to controls. Myocardial tissues from rats treated with WS and subjected to ischemia and reperfusion showed a decrease in these changes. The authors concluded that the results "emphasize the beneficial action of WS as a cardioprotective agent". In another similar investigation, Mohanty and coworkers[7] found that cardioprotection by WS is due to its antioxidant property and ability to attenuate ischemia-reperfusion-induced apoptosis.

El Kiki and coworkers[8] examined the effect of a Withania somnifera root extract on gamma radiation-induced cardiotoxicity in rats. Male albino rats treated with the vehicle for 7 days and exposed to gamma radiation (6 Gy) showed increased levels of serum urea and creatinine, CPK and LDH activities, as well as increased NO and MDA levels and decreased SOD in cardiac tissues compared to controls. Rats treated with WS (10 mg/kg, via tube) and exposed to gamma radiation reversed these changes.

Mohan and coworkers[9] investigated the cardioprotective effect of CardiPro against doxorubicin (DXR)-induced cardiotoxicity in mice. CardiPro is a polyherbal formulation containing Withania somnifera. Female Swiss albino mice treated with DXR (4 mg/kg/week, i.p.) for 4 weeks showed signs of cardiotoxicity: increased mortality, accumulation of ascitic fluid, decreased heart weight, decreased total antioxidant activity in heart tissue and histopathological changes in the heart. Mice treated with CardiPro (150 mg/kg, P.O.), twice a day for 7 weeks along with four injections of DXR showed a reversal of the effects of DXR.

References

1   Cardiovascular Diseases (CVDs). World Health Organization. https://www.who.int/en/news-room/fact-sheets/detail/cardiovascular-diseases-(cvds)

2   Heart Disease. Centers for Disease Control and Prevention. https://www.cdc.gov/heartdisease/facts.htm

3   Ipseeta Mohanty, Dharamvir Singh Arya, Amit Dinda, Keval Kishan Talwar, Sujata Joshi and Suresh Kumar Gupta. Mechanisms of cardioprotective effect of Withania somnifera in experimentally induced myocardial infarction. Basic and Clinical Pharmacology & Toxicology (2004) 94: 184-190.

4   Md. Ibrahim Khalil, Istiyak Ahmmed, Romana Ahmed, E. M. Tanvir, Rizwana Afroz, Sudip Paul, Siew Hua Gan, and Nadia Alam. Amelioration of isoproterenol-induced oxidative damage in rat myocardium by Withania somnifera leaf extract. BioMed Research International (20015) Article ID 624159, 10 pages.

5   A. Hamza, A. Amin, S. Daoud. The protective effect of a purified extract of Withania somnifera against doxorubicin-induced cardiac toxicity in rats. Cell Biol Toxicol (2008) 24: 63-73.

6   Suresh Kumar Gupta, Ipseeta Mohanty, Keval Krishan Talwar, Amit Dinda, Sujata Joshi, Pankaj Bansal, Amit Saxena and Dharamvir Singh Arya. Cardioprotection from ischemia and reperfusion injury by Withania somnifera: A hemodynamic, biochemical and histopathological assessment. Molecular and Cellular Biochemistry (2004) 260: 39-47.

7   Ipseeta Ray Mohanty, Dharamvir Singh Arya, Suresh Kumar Gupta. Withania somnifera provides cardioprotection and attenuates ischemia-reperfusion induced apoptosis. Clinical Nutrition (2008) 27: 635-642.

8   Shereen M. El Kiki, Heba H. Mansour and Lubna M. Anis. The modulatory role of Ashwagandha root extract on gamma-radiation-induced nephrotoxicity and cardiotoxicity in male albino rats. American Journal of Phytomedicine and Clinical Therapeutics (2014) 2 (5): 622-629.

9   I. K. Mohan, K. V. Kumar, M. U. R. Naidu, M. Khan, C. Sundaram. Protective effect of CardiPro against doxorubicin-induced cardiotoxicity in mice. Phytomedicine (2006) 13 (4): 222-229.

12 – Antidiabetic Activity

12.1 – Introduction

Diabetes is a chronic disease characterized by elevated blood glucose levels (hyperglycemia). It is caused by inadequate insulin production, ineffective use of insulin, or both. Insulin is a hormone produced by the pancreas. It enables cells to absorb glucose from the bloodstream. When insufficient or defective insulin is produced, glucose accumulates in the blood. Chronic hyperglycemia can cause serious damage to nerves, blood vessels, and organs such as the eyes, kidneys and heart.

There are three major types of diabetes: type 1, type 2 and gestational. In type 1, the pancreas produces little or no insulin. It is most often diagnosed in children, teens and young adults, and it accounts for less than 10% of the diabetic population. Treatment includes proper diet, exercise and daily insulin injections. Type 2 is caused by the body's ineffective use of insulin. The majority of the diabetic population belong to this category. Type 2 occurs most often in adults, but teens are increasingly being diagnosed with it. Treatment includes proper diet, exercise, and in many cases oral hypoglycemic agents and/or insulin. Gestational diabetes sometimes occurs in pregnant women.

An estimated 422 million people had diabetes globally in 2014[1]. According to a CDC report, 30.3 million Americans had diabetes in 2015 and it was the seventh leading cause of death[2]. A number of studies have examined the antidiabetic activity of Withania somnifera and the results are summarized below.

12.2 – Summary of Results

Anwer and coworkers[3] investigated the effect of an aqueous extract of Withania somnifera root (WS) on insulin sensitivity in non-insulin-dependent diabetes mellitus (NIDDM) rats. NIDDM was induced in albino Wistar pups (2 days old) by injecting a single dose of streptozotocin (100 mg/kg, i.p.) in citrate buffer. Diabetes was confirmed by measuring fasting blood glucose levels after 10 days ($\geq$ 200 mg/dl). Normal rat pups treated with citrate buffer served as controls. NIDDM rats showed an increased blood glucose level, HbA1c level and serum insulin level compared to controls. NIDDM rats treated with WS (200 or 400 mg/kg/day, P.O.) for 5 weeks showed a reversal of the changes observed in NIDDM rats. In NIDDM rats, the oral glucose tolerance test showed an increased blood glucose level with time and the high glucose level was maintained for 1 hour. Treatment with WS reduced the peak glucose level. In a subsequent investigation, Anwer and coworkers[4] showed that diabetes increased LPO and decreased the activities of GPx, GR, GST, SOD and CAT in pancreatic tissue compared to controls. NIDDM rats treated with WS showed a reversal of the changes observed in NIDDM rats.

Udayakumar and coworkers[5] investigated the antidiabetic effect of an ethanol (80%) extract of Withania somnifera roots (WSREt) and leaves (WSLEt) in diabetic rats. Glibenclamide, a common diabetic drug, was also tested for comparison. Adult male albino rats were injected with alloxan (150 mg/kg, i.p.) in saline to induce diabetes. Normal rats treated with saline served as controls. After 8 weeks of diabetes induction, the rats showed decreased body weight and liver glycogen, and increased urine sugar, blood glucose and HbA1c compared to controls. Diabetic rats treated with WSREt (100 or 200 mg/kg/day, via intragastric tube), WSLEt (100 or 200 mg/kg/day, via intragastric tube) or glibenclamide (0.6 mg/kg/day, P.O.) for 8 weeks showed a reversal of these changes. The effect of the extracts was comparable to glibenclamide. In another investigation, Udayakumar and coworkers[6] found decreased vitamin C and vitamin E in plasma, and decreased SOD, CAT, GPx, GSH and GST in kidney, heart and liver tissues of diabetic rats compared to controls. Diabetic rats treated with WSREt (100 or 200 mg/kg/day, via gastric tube), WSLEt (100 or 200 mg/kg/day, via gastric tube) or glibenclamide (0.6 mg/kg/day, P.O.) for 8 weeks showed a reversal of the above changes to near-control levels.

Sarangi and coworkers[7] examined the antidiabetic activity of an ethanol (80%) extract of Withania somnifera roots (WSREt) and leaves (WSLEt) in diabetic rats. Adult male albino rats were injected with streptozotocin (150 mg/kg, i.p.) in saline and diabetes was confirmed after a fortnight (blood glucose 250-300 mg/dl). Normal healthy rats treated with saline served as controls. Diabetic rats showed increased blood glucose (401 mg/dl) after 8 weeks compared to controls. Diabetic rats treated with WSREt (200 mg/kg/day, via intragastric tube or WSLEt (200 mg/kg/day, via intragastric tube) for 8 weeks showed decreased blood glucose compared to diabetic rats not treated with the extract.

Dayananda and coworkers[8] reported the antidiabetic effect of aqueous and alcoholic extracts of Withania somnifera in diabetic rats. Alloxan was injected (150 mg/kg, i.p.) and diabetes was confirmed after 72 hours. Diabetic rats treated with the aqueous or alcoholic extract of WS (250 mg/kg/day, P.O.) for 15 days showed decreased blood glucose levels compared to diabetic rats not treated with the extract.

Noshahr and coworkers[9] investigated the effect of Withania somnifera root (WS) powder on insulin resistance and inflammatory markers in fructose-fed rats. Male Wistar rats fed with fructose (10% W/V solution) along with a standard pellet diet for 8 weeks showed higher blood glucose levels, increased levels of insulin, TNF-α and IL-6 in plasma, and increased HOMA-R (an index of hepatic insulin resistance) compared to controls (rats fed a standard pellet diet and water). Rats treated with WS and fructose along with a standard pellet diet showed a reversal of these changes. The authors suggested that "WS may be suitable supplement for the prevention of diabetic complications".

Safhi and Anwer[10] studied the effect of an aqueous extract of Withania somnifera roots (WS) in type 2 diabetic rats. Diabetes was induced in albino Wistar rats (2 days old) by injecting streptozotocin (100 mg/kg, i.p.). Diabetic rats showed increased levels of blood glucose, glycosylated hemoglobin (HbA1c) and serum insulin, decreased KITT (insulin sensitivity index), and increased HOMA-R compared to controls (albino Wistar rats treated with citrate buffer). Diabetic rats treated with WS (200 or 400 mg/kg/day, P.O.) for 5 weeks showed a reversal of these changes. Also, diabetic rats treated with WS showed a significant improvement in glucose tolerance compared to untreated diabetic rats.

Nirupama and coworkers[11] investigated the hypoglycemic potential of various extracts of Ashwagandha roots. Ashwagandha root powder was extracted successively with petroleum ether, benzene, chloroform and ethanol. In vitro assays (glucose uptake by yeast cells, α-amylase inhibitory activity, glucose adsorption and diffusion) showed hypoglycemic activity of the extracts. The chloroform and ethanol extracts were more effective than others, and their hypoglycemic activity was also demonstrated by in vivo studies. These extracts prevented stress-induced hyperglycemia in male Wistar rats. The authors concluded that "Ashwagandha prevents either postprandial or stress induced hyperglycaemia by utilizing different mechanisms".

Bhattacharya and coworkers[12] reported that Trasina, an ayurvedic herbal formulation containing Ashwagandha, decreased streptozotocin (STZ)-induced hyperglycemia and attenuated the STZ-induced decrease in pancreatic islet SOD activity in rats.

Tekula and coworkers[13] examined the antidiabetic effect of Withaferin A (WA) in multiple low doses of streptozotocin (MLD-STZ)-induced type 1 diabetes mellitus (T1DM) in mice. T1DM was induced in male Swiss albino mice by administering STZ (40 mg/kg/day, i.p.) for 5 days. The T1DM mice showed the following changes compared to controls: decreased pancreatic weight, increased blood glucose levels, impaired glucose clearance, decreased plasma and tissue levels of insulin, oxidative and nitrosative stress, elevation of inflammatory cytokines, and destruction of beta cells. Mice treated with STZ and WA (2 or 10 mg/kg/day) concurrently for 5 days showed a reversal of the changes observed in T1DM mice.

A number of in vitro studies[14-16] have shown that Withania somnifera inhibits glycation, formation of advanced glycation products, and cross-linking of collagen incubated with glucose. One study showed that the effect of an ethanol extract of Withania somnifera roots was comparable to metformin, a known antiglycating agent.

Khalili[17] showed the antinociceptive effect of Ashwagandha on formalin-induced pain in diabetic rats (STZ-induced). Pradeep and coworkers[18] also showed that treatment of diabetic rats (STZ-induced) with an aqueous extract of Withania somnifera (100 mg/kg/day, P.O.) for 21 days reduced neuropathic pain.

Andallu and Radhika[19] studied the hypoglycemic, diuretic and hypocholesterolemic effects of Withania somnifera roots (WS) in human subjects. Mild NIDDM subjects were given WS (1000 mg) thrice daily or daonil (an oral hypoglycemic drug) for 30 days. Both groups showed a 12% reduction in blood sugar compared to their baseline. The WS group showed a decrease in serum potassium and an increase in urine sodium and urine volume. The WS group also showed a decrease in serum cholesterol, triglycerides, LDL and VLDL cholesterol, and a slight increase in HDL cholesterol. The treatment was well tolerated without any adverse side effects.

Usharani and coworkers[20] conducted a randomized, double-blind, placebo-controlled study to evaluate the effect of a highly standardized Withania somnifera extract (WS) on endothelial dysfunction and biomarkers of oxidative stress in type 2 diabetic patients maintained on metformin. 66 patients were randomized into three groups and respectively treated with 250 mg of WS, 500 mg of WS, or placebo twice daily for 12 weeks. 60 patients completed the study. The WS-treated groups showed significant improvements in endothelial function (decreased reflection index), biomarkers of oxidative stress (decreased malondialdehyde and increased nitric oxide and glutathione), systemic inflammation (reduction of high sensitivity C reactive proteins), lipid parameters (decreased total cholesterol, LDL cholesterol and triglycerides) and HbA1c levels. The treatment was well tolerated. The authors suggested that "W. somnifera could be further evaluated for its therapeutic role as an adjunctive in the management of diabetes mellitus associated with endothelial dysfunction".

Upadhyay and coworkers[21] examined the effect of Ashwagandha (ASH) and Shilajit (SH) extracts in NIDDM patients. 32 subjects with early diagnosed type 2 diabetes were treated with two capsules (250 mg ASH + 250 mg SH per capsule) in the morning and two in the evening for 4 weeks. At the end of the therapy, the subjects showed reduced blood sugar, total cholesterol (TC), LDL and VLDL cholesterol, and TC/HDL.

References

1 Diabetes. World Health Organization. https://www.who.int/news-room/fact-sheets/detail/diabetes

2 New CDC report: More than 100 million Americans have diabetes or pre diabetes. Centers for Disease Control and Prevention. https://www.cdc.gov/media/releases/2017/p0718-diabetes-report.html

3 Tarique Anwer, Manju Sharma, Krishna Kolappa Pillai and Muzaffar Iqbal. Effect of Withania somnifera on insulin sensitivity in non-insulin-dependent diabetes mellitus rats. Basic & Clinical Pharmacology & Toxicology (2008) 102: 498-503.

4 Tarique Anwer, Manju Sharma, Krishna Kolappa Pillai and Gyas Khan. Protective effect of Withania somnifera against oxidative stress and pancreatic β-cell damage in type 2 diabetic rats. Drug Research (2012) 69 (6): 1095-1101.

5 Rajangam Udayakumar, Sampath Kasthurirengan, Thankaraj Salammal Mariashibu, Manoharan Rajesh, Vasudevan Ramesh Anbazhagan, Sei Chang Kim, Andy Ganapathi and Chang Won Choi. Hypoglycaemic and Hypolipidaemic effect of Withania somnifera root and leaf extracts on alloxan-induced diabetic rats. Int. J. Mol. Sci (2009) 10: 2367-2382.

6 Rajangam Udayakumar, Sampath Kasthurirengan, Ayyappa Vasudevan, Thankaraj Salammal Mariashibu, Jesudass Joseph Sahaya Rayan, Chang Won Choi, Andy Ganapathi, Sei Chang Kim. Antioxidant effect of dietary supplement Withania somnifera L. reduce blood glucose levels in alloxan-induced diabetic rats. Plant Foods Hum Nutr (2010) 65: 91-98.

7 Sarangi, A., Jena, S., Sarangi, A. K. and Swain, B. Anti-diabetic effects of Withania somnifera root and leaf extracts on streptozotocin induced diabetic rats. Journal of Cell and Tissue Research (2013) 13 (1): 3597-3601.

8 K. S. Dayananda, S. M. Gopinath, Shwetha C. P, Ajay Mandal. Hypoglycemic activity of aqueous, and ethanolic extracts of Tinosora cordifolia, Phyllanthus emblica, Gymnema sylvesre and Withania somnifera in alloxan induced diabetic rats. International Journal of Indigenous

Medicinal plants (2014) 47(2): 1627-1632.

9 Zahra Samadi Noshahr, Mohammad Reza Shahraki, Hassan Ahmadvand, Davood Nourabadi, Alireza Nakhaei. Protective effects of Withania somnifera root on inflammatory markers and insulin resistance in fructose-fed rats. Reports of Biochemistry & Molecular Biology (2015) 3 (2): 62 – 67.

10 Mohammed M. A Safhi, Tarique Anwer. Comparative analysis of Withania somnifera and Rhus coriaria on hyperglycemia and insulin sensitivity in type 2 diabetic rats. Journal of Jazan University (2011) 1 (1): 1-14.

11 R. Nirupama, M. Devaki, M. Nirupama and H. N. Yajurvedi. In vitro and in vivo studies on the hypoglycaemic potential of Ashwagandha (Withania somnifera) root. Pharma Science Monitor (2014) 5(3) spul1: 45-48.

12 Bhattacharya SK, Satyan KS, Chakrabarti A. Effect of Trasina, an Ayurvedic herbal formulation, on pancreatic islet superoxide dismutase activity in hyperglycaemic rats. Indian J Exp Biol (1997) 35(3): 297-9.

13 Sravani Tekula, Amit Khurana, Pratibha Anchi, Chandraiah Godugu. Withaferin A attenuates multiple low doses of streptozotocin (MLD-STD) induced type 1 diabetes. Biomedicine & Pharmacotherapy (2018) 106: 1428–1440.

14 Pon Velayutham Anandh Babu, Adikesavan Gokulakrishnan, Rajendra Dhandayuthbani, Dowlath Ameethkhan, Chandrasekara Vimal Pradeep Kumar, Md Iqbal Niyas Ahmad. Protective effect of Withania somnifera (solanaceae) on collagen glycation and cross-linking. Comparative Biochemistry and Physiology Part B: Biochemistry and Molecular Biology (2007) 147 (2): 308-313.

15 Nadeem Khan, Ragini Gothalwal, N.M. Shrivastava and Savita Shrivastava. Evaluate the effect of Withania somnifera methanolic extracts as in vitro antiglycating agents. Octa Journal of Bioscience (2014) 2 (1): 13-17.

16 Nadeem Khan and Ragini Gothalwal. An anti-glycating property roots ethanol and methanol extracts of Withania somnifera on in vitro glycation of elastin protein. International Journal of Current Microbiology and Applied Sciences (2015) 4 (9): 899-908.

17 Mohsen Khalili. The effect of oral administration of Withania somnifera root on formalin-induced pain in diabetic rats. Basic and Clinical Neuroscience (2009) 1 (1): 29-31.

18 Pradeep S., Prem Kumar N, Deepak Kumar Khajuria, Srinivas Rao G. Preclinical evaluation of antinociceptive effect of Withania somnifera (Ashwagandha) in diabetic peripheral neuropathic rat models. Pharamcologyonline (2010) 2: 283-298.

19 B Andallu & B Radhika. Hypoglycemic, diuretic and hypocholesterolemic effect of Winter cherry (Withania somnifera, Dunal) root. Indian Journal of Experimental Biology (2000) 38: 607-609.

20 Pingali Usharani, Nishat Fatima, Chiranjeevi Uday Kumar, P. V. Kishan. Evaluation of a highly standardized Withania somnifera extract on endothelial dysfunction and biomarkers of oxidative stress in patients with type 2 diabetes mellitus: A randomized, double blind, placebo controlled study. International Journal of Ayurveda and Pharma Research (2014) 2 (3): 22-32.

21 Avinash K Upadhyay, Kumar Kaushal, Mishra Harishankar. Effects of combination of Shilajit extract and Ashwagandha (Withania somnifera) on fasting blood sugar and lipid profile. Journal of Pharmacy Research (2009) 2 (5): 897-899.

13 – Liver and Kidney Protective Activities

13.1 – Introduction

The liver is the largest internal organ of the body and weighs about 3.5 lbs. It is located in the upper right-hand portion of the abdominal cavity below the diaphragm. The liver performs many vital functions such as the production of bile; metabolism of carbohydrates; conversion of excess glucose to glycogen; storage of glycogen, vitamins and minerals; synthesis of plasma proteins; and detoxification and elimination of toxic substances[1]. Causes of liver diseases include viruses (e.g. hepatitis A, B and C), drugs, poisons and excessive use of alcohol.

The human body has two kidneys, each about the size of a fist. They are located on either side of the spine below the rib cage. The kidneys are highly specialized organs that play an important role in regulating the volume and composition of extracellular fluid. They maintain a stable internal environment by selectively excreting appropriate amounts of various substances according to specific bodily needs. The kidneys perform a variety of functions that include balancing fluid levels, elimination of waste products and regulation of blood plasma ion concentration. They also produce hormones that regulate blood pressure, help produce red blood cells and promote bone health[2]. Kidneys are susceptible to various diseases, and most kidney problems are associated with diseases such as diabetes and hypertension. A number of investigations have been conducted to examine the liver and kidney protective activities of Withania somnifera and the results are summarized below.

13.2 – Summary of Results

Bhattacharya and coworkers[3] investigated the effect of Withania somnifera glycowithanolides (WSG) on iron-induced hepatotoxicity in rats. Adult male Wistar rats treated with saline for ten days followed by a single dose of ferrous sulfate (2.5 mg/kg, i.p.) showed increased hepatic LPO and serum ALAT, ASAT and LDH compared to the saline-treated group. Rats treated with WSG (10-50 mg/kg/day, P.O.) for 10 days followed by a single dose of ferrous sulfate (2.5 mg/kg, i.p.) showed a mitigation of these changes. The effect of WSG (50 mg/kg) was comparable to the effect of silymarin (20 mg/kg), a standard hepatoprotective agent.

Akbarsha and coworkers[4] reported that Withania somnifera root powder (WS) reversed the liver and kidney damage in rats induced by carbendazim (methyl-2-benzimidazole carbamate, MBC), a widely used fungicide. Male albino Wistar rats treated with a single bolus dose of MBC (400 mg/kg) showed severe histopathological liver and kidney lesions compared to controls. Rats treated with a single dose of MBC (400 mg/kg) followed by treatment with WS (250 mg/kg/day, via oral gavage) for 48 days showed a liver and kidney histoarchitecture similar to controls.

Ganguly and coworkers[5] examined the hepatoprotective effect of withasteroid metal conjugates of Withania somnifera on paracetamol-induced hepatotoxicity in rats. A dried powder of Withania somnifera roots and leaves was extracted with hot water. The dried residue (WSE) was dissolved in a minimum volume of water and passed successively through weak and strong cation exchange resins. The excluded fractions WSE/excluded-I and WSE/excluded-II were used in the study. Albino rats treated with paracetamol (500 mg/kg/day, P.O.) for 7 days showed increased liver weight and increased serum SGOT, SGPT, ALP and bilirubin as well as increased LPO and decreased GSH, SOD and CAT in the liver homogenate compared to controls. Rats treated with WSE (200 mg/kg/day, P.O.)+paracetamol or WSE/excluded-I (100 mg/kg/day, P.O.)+paracetamol for 7 days showed a reversal of the changes induced by paracetamol. WSE/excluded-I was more effective than WSE. Rats treated with WSE/excluded-II (100 mg/kg/day, P.O.)+paracetamol showed marginal effects on the paracetamol-induced changes. The authors concluded that "Based on the above findings it is postulated that metal ions in conjugation with the withasteroids have a profound bearing on the true bioactive principles of the adaptogenic Withania somnifera standardized extract(s)".

Malik and coworkers[6] demonstrated the hepatoprotective effect of an aqueous extract of Withania somnifera roots (WS) in mice. Female Swiss albino mice treated with paracetamol (500 mg/kg/day, via oral gavage) 6 days a week for 28 days showed increased serum ALT, AST, ALP, bilirubin and proteins as well as increased LPO and decreased GSH, CAT, GR and GPx in the liver compared to controls. Mice treated with paracetamol (500 mg/kg/day, via oral gavage), followed by WS (500 mg/kg/day via oral gavage) 6 days a week for 28 days showed a reversal of these changes. Liver sections of the paracetamol-treated group showed major histological changes compared to controls, whereas mice treated with paracetamol and WS showed normal architecture. The authors concluded that "this study signifies that Withania somnifera root extract shows hepatoprotective effect through its antioxidant potential on paracetamol induced liver damage in mice. However, further studies are required to elucidate the molecular mechanisms involved in order to support the clinical use of this extract".

Elberry and coworkers[7] evaluated the effect of a methanol extract of Withania somnifera aerial parts (WS) on carbon tetrachloride (CCl_4)-induced hepatotoxicity in rats. Male Wistar rats treated with CCl_4 showed increased serum AST, ALT, ALP and LDH as well as increased LPO and decreased GPx, GR, GST and GSH in the liver compared to controls. Rats treated with CCl_4 +WS showed a reversal of these changes. Liver sections of the CCl_4 group showed major histopathological changes compared to controls, whereas the CCl_4+WS group was similar to controls.

Sharma and coworkers[8] investigated the hepatoprotective potential of a hydromethanolic (20:80) extract of Withania somnifera roots (WS) in mice. Swiss albino mice treated with lead nitrate (20 mg/kg/day) for 42 days showed increased hepatic LPO and decreased SOD, CAT, GST, GSH and protein compared to controls. Mice treated with lead nitrate (200 mg/kg/day)+WS (500 mg/kg/day) for 42 days showed a reversal of these changes. Liver sections of mice treated with lead nitrate showed major histopathological alterations compared to controls, whereas mice treated with lead nitrate+WS showed only minor histopathological alterations.

Sabina and coworkers[9] reported the hepatoprotective effect of Withania somnifera in paracetamol-treated rats. Rats treated with a single dose of paracetamol (900 mg/kg, i.p.) showed increased serum ALT, AST, ASP, total bilirubin and protein and decreased SOD, CAT and GSH compared to controls. Rats treated with a single dose of paracetamol followed by WS (500 or 1000 mg/kg, P.O.) showed a reversal of these changes. Liver sections of rats treated with paracetamol showed major histological changes compared to controls, whereas rats treated with paracetamol+WS showed no visible histological changes.

Vedi and coworkers[10] investigated the effect of Withania somnifera root on bromobenzene-induced hepatotoxicity in rats. Wistar albino rats treated with a single dose of bromobenzene (10 mmol/kg in 0.1 ml coconut oil) showed the following changes compared to controls:

- increased liver weight and increased serum AST, ALP, total bilirubin, direct bilirubin and albumin

- increased LPO and depleted plasma and liver antioxidants
- decreased liver mitochondrial enzymes (TCA cycle and respiratory enzymes)
- increased serum TNF-α, IL-1β and VEGF

Rats treated with WS (250 or 500 mg/kg/day, P.O.) for 8 days followed by treatment with bromobenzene showed attenuation of the changes induced by bromobenzene. Histopathological studies of the liver sections of rats treated with bromobenzene showed massive changes compared to controls. Rats treated with WS+bromobenzene showed almost control architecture.

Mansour and Hafez[11] examined the hepatoprotective activity of an alcohol extract of Withania somnifera roots in rats. Hepatotoxicity was induced by ionizing radiation. Male albino rats treated with distilled water for 7 days and exposed to a single dose of gamma-irradiation (6-Gy) showed increased serum AST, ALT, ALP and GST as well as increased hepatic LPO, NO(x) and HO-1 activity and decreased hepatic SOD, GSHPx and GSH compared to controls. Rats treated with WS (100 mg/kg/day, via gavage) for 7 days and exposed to a single dose of gamma-irradiation (6-Gy) showed a mitigation of the changes induced by gamma-irradiation. The authors concluded that "these observations suggest that WS could be developed as a potential preventive drug for ionizing radiation induced hepatotoxicity disorders via enhancing the antioxidant activity and induction of HO-1".

Gopinath and coworkers[12] showed the hepatoprotective effect of a Withania somnifera root extract (WS) against chlorpyrifos (CPF)-induced liver damage in mice. CPF (O,O-diethyl-3,5,6-trichloro-pyridyl phospothionate) is a pesticide. Swiss albino mice treated with CPF for 28 days showed increased serum AST and ALT, increased liver LPO and decreased liver antioxidants compared to controls. Mice treated with WS+CPF for 28 days showed decreased serum AST and ALT, decreased liver LPO and increased antioxidants compared to the CPF-only group.

Al-Awthan and coworkers[13] found that an aqueous extract of Withania somnifera (WS) attenuated hepatotoxicity induced by dimethoate (DM) in guinea pigs. DM is an organophosphorus insecticide. Male guinea pigs treated with DM (14 mg/kg/day, P.O.) for 21 days showed increased serum AST, ALT and ALP compared to controls. Guinea pigs treated with WS (100 mg/kg/day, P.O.) followed by DM (14 mg/kg/day, P.O.) for 21 days showed decreased levels of serum AST, ALT and ALP compared to the DM-only group. Liver sections of the DM-only group showed major histopathological alterations compared to controls, whereas in the WS+DM group the changes were minor.

Harikrishnan and coworkers[14] reported that treating male albino Wistar rats with NH_4Cl (100 mg/kg/day, i.p), thrice a week for 8 weeks increased serum AST, ALT and ALP and increased blood ammonia, urea, LPO and HP compared to controls. Rats treated with NH_4Cl (100 mg/kg/day, i.p) and an ethanol (95%) extract of Withania somnifera roots (500 mg/kg, via intragastric gavage) thrice a week for 8 weeks showed no significant difference in the above parameters compared to controls.

Bhattacharjee and coworkers[15] examined the effect of an aqueous extract of Withania somnifera root (WS) on carbofuran-induced hepatotoxicity in fish. Carbofuran (2,3-dihydro-2,2-dimethyl-7-benzofuranyl methylcarbamate) is one of the most toxic carbamate pesticides. Fish treated with carbofuran for 30 days showed increased serum SGPT, bilirubin, glucose and hemoglobin compared to controls. Fish treated with carbofuran for 30 days followed by treatment with WS for 6 weeks showed decreased serum SGPT bilirubin, glucose and hemoglobin compared to the carbofuran-only group. Liver sections of the carbofuran-only group showed major histopathological changes compared to controls, whereas the carbofuran+WS group showed only minor changes.

Sharma and coworkers[16] examined the therapeutic efficacy of a methanol (90%) extract of Withania somnifera roots in the mitigation of lead nitrate-induced nephrotoxicity in mice. Male Swiss albino mice treated with lead nitrate (20 mg/kg) showed increased LPO and decreased kidney SOD, CAT, GST, GSH and proteins compared to controls. Mice treated with the extract and lead nitrate showed a reduction of the changes induced by lead nitrate. Kidney sections of the lead nitrate-only group showed major histological changes compared to controls, whereas the extract+lead nitrate group showed only minor changes.

Kushwaha and coworkers[17] reported the nephroprotective activity of an aqueous extract of Withania somnifera roots (WS) on gentamicin-induced nephrotoxicity in rats. Wistar albino rats treated with saline for 30 days and injected with gentamicin during the last 5 days (40 mg/kg/day, i.p.) showed increased serum BUN and creatinine compared to controls. Rats treated with WS (500 mg/kg/day, P.O.) for 30 days and injected with gentamicin during the last five days showed a reduction of these changes. In another study, Kushwaha[18] showed that 30 days of WS treatment offered better nephroprotection than 10 days of WS treatment for gentamicin-induced nephrotoxicity in rats.

Shimmi and coworkers[19] examined the effect of Withania somnifera (WS) on gentamicin-induced nephrotoxicity in rats. Wistar albino rats given a basal diet for 22 days and injected with gentamicin (100 mg/kg/day, S.C.) during the last 8 days showed increased kidney weight, serum urea and creatinine compared to controls. Rats treated with WS (500 mg/kg/day, P.O.) for 22 days along with the basal diet and injected with gentamicin showed decreased kidney weight, serum urea and creatinine compared to the gentamicin-only group. A similar investigation[20] showed that gentamicin reduced serum potassium ion levels, and pretreatment with Ashwagandha mitigated the effect of gentamicin.

Govindappa and coworkers[21] examined the effect of an alcohol extract of Withania somnifera roots (WS) on gentamicin (GM)-induced renal lesions in rats. Male Wistar rats treated with GM (80 mg/kg/day, i.p.) for 8 days showed the following changes compared to controls: reduced body weight and increased kidney weight, increased BUN and serum concentrations of creatinine, albumin, gamma-glutamyl transferase, ALP, ALT, and AST, increased serum electrolytes (K^+ and Ca^{2+}), increased LPO, and decreased SOD and GSH. Rats treated with WS (500 mg/kg/day, P.O.) for 13 days followed by simultaneous treatment with GM and WS (nephroprotective group) for 7 days showed a reversal of the changes observed in the GM-only group. Also, rats treated with GM for 8 days followed by WS treatment on days 9-21 showed a reversal of the changes observed in the GM-only group. The GM-only group showed swollen kidneys and major histopathological changes. The nephroprotective group showed only minor changes.

El Kiki and coworkers[22] examined the effect of a Withania somnifera root extract (WS) on gamma radiation-induced nephrotoxicity in rats. Male albino rats treated with the vehicle for 7 days and exposed to a single dose of gamma radiation showed increased serum urea, creatinine, CPK and LDH as well as increased LPO and NO and decreased SOD and GSH in kidney tissues compared to controls. Rats treated with WS (100 mg/kg/day) for 7 days and exposed to gamma radiation showed a reversal of these changes.

References

1   Premalatha Balachandran, Rajgopal Govindarajan. "Hepatic disorders" in Scientific Basis for Ayurvedic Therapies. Edited by Lakshmi Chandra Mishra. CRC Press, Boca Raton, FL 2004.
2   Raghavendra Mallikarjun, M J Vidya, Functions of kidney and artificial kidneys. International Journal of Innovative Research in Electrical, Electronics, Instrumentation and Control Engineering (2013) 1 (1): 1-5.
3   A. Bhattacharya, M. Ramanathan, S. Ghosal and S. K. Bhattacharya. Effect 0f

Withania somnifera glycowithanolides on iron-induced hepatotoxicity in rats. Phytother Res (2000) 14: 568-570.

4   M. A. Akbarsha, S. Vijendrakumar, B. Kadalmani, R. Girija and A. Faridha. Curative property of Withania somnifera Dunal root in the context of carbendazim-induced histopathological changes in the liver and kidney of rat. Phytomedicine (2000) 7(6): 499-507.

5   Partha Ganguly, Amartya K Gupta, Upal K Majumder, Shibnath Ghosal. Hepatoprotective and antioxidant effects of naturally occurring withasteroid metal ion conjugates of Withania somnifera in paracetamol induced hepatotoxicity in rats. Pharmacologyonline (2009) 1: 1049-1056.

6   Tabarak Malik, Devendra Kumar Pandey and Nitu Dogra. Ameliorative potential of aqueous root extract of Withania somnifera against paracetamol induced liver damage in mice. Pharmacologia (2013) 89-94.

7   Ahmed A. Elberry, Fathalla M. Harraz, Salah A. Ghareib, Ayman A. Nagy, Salah A. Gabr, Mansour I. Suliaman and Essam Abdel-Sattar. Antihepatotoxic effect of Marrubium vulgare and Withania somnifera extracts on carbon tetrachloride-induced hepatotoxicity in rats. Journal of Basic and Clinical Pharmacy (2010) 1(4): 247-254.

8   Veena Sharma, Sadhana Sharma, Pracheta, Shatruhan Sharma. Lead induced hepatotoxicity in male Swiss albino mice: The protective potential of the hydromethanolic extract of Withania somnifera. International Journal of Pharmaceutical Sciences Review and Research (2011) 7 (2): 116-121.

9   Evan Prince Sabina, Mahaboobkhan Rasool, Mahima Vedi, Dhanalakshmi Navaneethan, Meenakshi Ravichander, Poornima Parthasarathy, Sarah Rachel Thella. Hepatoprotective and antioxidant potential of Withania somnifera against paracetamol-induced liver damage in rats. International Journal of Pharmacy and Pharmaceutical Sciences (2013) 5(2): 648-651.

10   Mahima Vedi, Mahaboobkhan Rasool, Evan Prince Sabina. Amelioration of bromobenzene hepatotoxicity by Withania somnifera pretreatment: Role of mitochondrial oxidative stress. Toxicology Reports (2014) 1: 629-638.

11   Heba Hosny Mansour, Hafez Farouk Hafez. Protective effect of Withania somnifera against radiation-induced hepatotoxicity in rats. Ecotoxicology and Environmental Safety (2012) 80: 14-19.

12   G. Gopinath, S. Uvarajan and A. Tamizselvi. Chlorpyrifos-induced oxidative stress and tissue damage in the liver of Swiss albino mice: the protective antioxidative role of root extract of Withania somnifera. IJIRST (2014) 1(6): 100-104.

13   Yahya S. Al-Awthan, Samira M. Hezar, Aisha M. Al-Zubairi and Faten A. Al-Hemiri. Effects of aqueous extract of Withania somnifera on some liver biochemical and histopathological parameters in male guinea pigs. Pakistan Journal of Biological Sciences (2014) 17 (4): 504-510.

14   B. Harikrishnan, P. Subramanian and S. Subash. Effect of Withania somnifera root powder on the levels of circulatory lipid peroxidation and liver markers enzymes in chronic hyperammonemia. E-Journal of Chemistry (2008) 5 (4): 872-877.

15   Soma Bhattacharjee, Prakriti Verma, Arun Kumar, Dharmendra Kumar Sinha and A. Nath. Role of Withania somnifera against carbofuran induced hepatotoxicity of fish, Clarias batrachus. J. Inland Fish. Soc. India (2008) 40 (2):50-55.

16   Veena Sharma, Sadhana Sharma, Pracheta, Ritu Paliwal, Shatruhan Sharma. Therapeutic efficacy of Withania somnifera root extract in the regulation of lead nitrate induced nephrotoxicity in Swiss albino mice. Journal of pharmacy research (2011) 4 (3): 755-758.

17   Vimlesh Kushwaha, Monica Sharma, Pinki Vishwakarma, Manish Saini,

Kuldeep Saxena. Biochemical assessment of nephroprotective and nephrocurative activity of Withania somnifera on gentamicin induced nephrotoxicity in experimental rats. International Journal of research in Medical Sciences (2016) 4 (1): 298-302.

18 Vimlesh Kushwaha. Nephroprotection of Withania somnifera root extract against gentamicin induced nephrotoxicity: a histological evaluation in experimental Wistar rats. International Journal of Basic & Clinical Pharmacology (2019) 8 (10): 2297-2303.

19 Sadia Choudhury Shimmi, Nasim Jahan, Nayma Sultana. Effect of Ashwagandha (Withania somnifera) root extract against gentamicin induced changes of serum urea and creatinine levels in rats. J Bangladesh Soc Physiol (2011) 6 (2): 84-89.

20 Sadia Choudhury Shimmi, Nasim Jahan, Nayma Sultan. Effects of Ashwagandha (Withania somnifera somnifera) root extract against gentamicin induced changes of serum electrolytes in rats. J Bangladesh Soc Physiol (2012) 7 (1):29-35.

21 Prem Kumar Govindappa, Vidhi Gautam, Syamantak Mani Tripathi, Yash Pal Sahni, Hallur Lakshmana Shetty Raghavendra. Effect of Withania somnifera on gentamicin induced renal lesions in rats. Revista Brasileira de Farmacognosia (2019) 29: 234 – 240.

22 Shereen M. El Kiki, Heba H. Mansour and Lubna M. Anis. The modulatory role of Ashwagandha root extract on gamma-radiation-induced nephrotoxicity and cardiotoxicity in male albino rats. American Journal of Phytomedicine and Clinical Therapeutics (2014) 2 (5): 622-629.

14 – Thyroid Protective Activity

14.1 – Introduction

The thyroid gland, responsible for regulating a wide range of physiological activities, is one of the most important endocrine organs. It is located in the middle of the lower neck, just above the collar bone. The thyroid gland produces the hormones thyroxine (T4) and triiodothyronine (T3) on stimulation by thyroid stimulating hormone (TSH) released from the pituitary gland. Approximately 90% of thyroid hormone production is T4, which is inactive, and approximately 10% is T3, which is active. Some of the T4 is metabolized to T3 in the liver.

Overproduction of the thyroid hormones leads to a condition known as hyperthyroidism and underproduction causes hypothyroidism[1]. Thyroid disorders are among the most common endocrine disorders worldwide. An estimated 20 million Americans have some form of thyroid disease[2]. Some studies have shown beneficial effects of Withania somnifera in the management of hypothyroidism and the results are summarized below.

14.2 – Summary of Results

Panda and Kar[3] examined the effect of an aqueous extract of Withania somnifera roots (WS) on thyroid hormone concentrations in mice. Adult male Swiss albino mice treated with WS (1.4 g/kg/day, gastric intubation) for 20 days showed increased serum concentrations of T3 and T4 as well as decreased LPO and increased activities of SOD and CAT in the liver. The authors concluded that "These findings reveal that the ashwagandha root extract stimulates thyroid activity and also enhances the antiperoxidation of hepatic tissue". A similar study[4] found that treating Swiss albino female mice with WS (1.4 g/kg/day, gastric intubation) for 20 days increased serum T4 without a significant change in T3. A later investigation[5] examined the combined effects of Withania somnifera roots (WS), Guggulu (G) and Bauhinia purpurea bark (BP) on thyroid function in mice. Adult female Swiss mice treated with WS (1.4 g/kg/day) + G (0.2 g/kg/day) + BP (2.5 mg/kg/day) by gastric intubation for 30 days showed increased serum T3 and T4, increased hepatic SOD and CAT, and no significant change in LPO. The authors suggested that "These plant extracts might be used to formulate a drug for the treatment of hypothyroidism".

Jatwa and Kar[6] reported that the administration of dexamethasone to adult Swiss albino female mice to induce type 2 diabetes also decreased the serum levels of T3 and T4. Administering metformin (antidiabetic drug) along with dexamethasone reversed the diabetic conditions but further decreased serum T4, indicating severe hypothyroidism. Administering an ethanol extract of Withania somnifera roots along with dexamethasone and metformin increased serum T3 and T4 to normal levels.

Abdel-Wahhab and coworkers[7] investigated the effect of a methanol extract of Ashwagandha roots (AME) on propylthiouracil-induced hypothyroidism in rats. Male albino rats treated with propylthiouracil (0.5% w/v) in drinking water for 6 weeks showed the following changes compared to controls (rats not given propylthiouracil):

- increased body weight
- increased serum TSH and decreased T3 (total and free) and T4 (total and free)
- increased serum glucose and IL-6 and decreased IL-10
- decreased blood hemoglobin
- increased hepatic and renal MDA and NO and decreased GSH, GPx and Na^+/K^+-ATPase

Rats treated with propylthiouracil for 6 weeks followed by treatment with AME (500 mg/kg/day) or an antihypothyroidism drug for one month reversed the changes induced by propylthiouracil. Thyroid glands from rats treated with propylthiouracil showed major histological changes compared to controls, whereas rats from the propylthiouracil+AME group showed only minor changes.

The authors concluded that "Ashwagandha methanolic extract treatment improves thyroid function by ameliorating thyroid hormones and by preventing oxidative stress".

Gannon and coworkers[8] conducted a placebo-controlled, randomized clinical trial in which an extract of Withania somnifera was used to improve cognitive function in patients with bipolar disorder. Patients treated with the extract showed improved thyroid indices (TSH, T4 and T3).

Sharma and coworkers[9] conducted a randomized, double-blind, placebo-controlled clinical trial to evaluate the efficacy and safety of an aqueous extract of Withania somnifera root in subclinical hypothyroid patients. 50 subjects with elevated levels of serum TSH (4.5-10 μIU/L) were randomized into a treatment group (n=25) and a placebo group (n=25). The subjects in the treatment group were given 300 mg of the extract in capsules twice a day for 8 weeks. The placebo group received placebo capsules. Levels of serum TSH, T3 and T4 were measured at baseline, week 4 and week 8. Four subjects (two from the treatment group and two from the placebo group) withdrew from the study. The treatment group showed decreased TSH and increased T3 and T4 compared to the placebo group. Treatment with the extract helped to normalize thyroid indices. Only a few subjects reported mild and temporary adverse side effects.

References

1   What is the thyroid? The American Association of Endocrine Surgeons Patient Education Site.
    https://collectedmed.com/index.php/article/article/demo_article_display/7561/83/1/1

2   General Information/Press Room, American Thyroid Association.
    https://www.thyroid.org/media-main/press-room/

3   Sunanda Panda and Anand Kar. Changes in thyroid hormone concentrations after administration of Ashwagandha root extract to adult male mice. J. Pharma. Pharmacol (1998) 50: 1065-1068.

4   S. Panda, A. Kar. Withania somnifera and Bauhinia purpurea in the regulation of circulating thyroid hormone concentrations in female mice. Journal of Ethnopharmacology (1999) 67: 233-239.

5   Sunanda Panda and Anand Kar. Combined effects of Ashwagandha, Guggulu and Bauhinia extracts in the regulation of thyroid function and on lipid peroxidation in mice. Pharm. Pharmacol. Commun (2000) 6: 141-143.

6   Rameshwar Jatwa and Anand Kar. Amelioration of metformin-induced hypothyroidism by Withania somnifera and Bauhinia purpurea extracts in type 2 diabetic mice. Phytotherapy Research (2009) 23: 1140-1145.

7   Khaled G. Abdel-Wahhab, Hagar H. Mourad. Fathia A. Mannaa. Fatma A. Morsy, Laila K. Hassan. Rehab F. Taher. Role of ashwagandha methanolic extract in the regulation of thyroid profile in hypothyroidism modeled rats. Molecular Biology Reports (2019) 46: 3637-3649.

8   Jessica M. Gannon, Paige E. Forrest, K. N. Roy Chengappa. Subtle changes in thyroid indices during a placebo-controlled study of an extract of Withania somnifera in persons with bipolar disorder. Journal of Ayurveda & Integrative Medicine (2014) 5 (4): 241-245.

9   Ashok Kumar Sharma, Indraneel Basu and Siddarth Singh. Efficacy and safety of Ashwagandha root extract in subclinical hypothyroid patients: A double-blind, randomized placebo-controlled trial. The Journal of Alternative and Complementary Medicine (2017) 0 (0): 1-6.

15 – Antiulcer Activity

15.1 – Introduction

Peptic ulcer disease (gastric and duodenal) is one of the most common disorders of the gastrointestinal tract[1]. Each year, more than half a million new cases are observed and more than one million people are hospitalized. An estimated 25 million Americans are affected by peptic ulcer disease in their lifetime. The two major causes of peptic ulcer disease are Helicobacter pylori infection and the long-term use of nonsteroidal anti-inflammatory drugs (NSAIDs) such as aspirin and ibuprofen[2]. Therapy for H. pylori infection includes antibiotics to kill the bacteria, proton pump inhibitors or histamine blockers to reduce stomach acid, and bismuth-containing agents to protect the stomach and duodenal lining. Treatment for NSAID-induced disease typically involves proton pump inhibitors or histamine blockers[3]. Among Ayurvedic herbal treatments, Withania somnifera is popular. A number of investigations have been done to evaluate the antiulcer effect of Withania somnifera and the results from some studies are summarized below.

15.2 – Summary of Results

Singh and coworkers[4] examined the antiulcer effect of an alcohol extract of Withania somnifera defatted seeds (WS) in rats subjected to cold stress, restraint stress, or treated with aspirin. Adult albino rats treated with WS (100 mg/kg, i.p.) and subjected to cold restraint stress for 2 hours at 4 °C, restraint stress for 18 hours, or treated with aspirin (200 mg/kg, i.p.) showed a decreased incidence of ulcer and a decreased mean ulcer index compared to rats treated with saline and subjected to stress or aspirin treatment.

Bhattacharya and coworkers[5] investigated the antiulcer activity of a methanol-water (1:1) extract of Withania somnifera root (SG-1) and an equimolecular combination of sitoindosides VII, VIII and Withaferin A (SG-2) in rats subjected to restraint stress. Rats treated with SG-1 or SG-2 (50 and 100 mg/kg/day, P.O.) for 4 days and subjected to restraint stress showed a decreased incidence and severity of ulcers compared to rats subjected to stress without SG-1 or SG-2 treatment. SG-2 was slightly more effective than SG-1.

Singh and coworkers[6] studied the effect of a withanolide-free aqueous fraction (BF) from Withania somnifera root against immobilization-induced gastric ulceration in rats. Charles Foster rats treated with BF (12.5-100 mg/kg/day, P.O.) for 15 days and subjected to immobilization stress for 5 hours on day 15 showed a dose-dependent decrease in ulcer incidence and ulcerogenic index compared to rats subjected to stress without BF treatment.

Bhattacharya and Muruganandan[7] examined the effect of an extract of Withania somnifera root (WS) on gastric ulceration induced by footshock stress. Adult male Wistar rats treated with WS (25 and 50 mg/kg/day, P.O.) and subjected to mild, unpredictable footshocks for 21 days showed a decreased incidence and severity of gastric ulcers compared to rats subjected to footshocks without WS treatment.

Bhatnagar and coworkers[8] reported the antiulcer activity of a methanol extract of Withania somnifera root (WS) against stress plus pyloric ligation-induced gastric ulcers in rats. Pyloric ligation was done only for the collection of gastric juice. Adult Wistar albino rats were treated with the vehicle (control), subjected to swim stress (5 h/day), or treated with WS (100 mg/kg/day, P.O.) and subjected to swim stress (5 h/day) for 15 days. Pyloric ligation was performed on the 16th day. Compared to controls, rats subjected to swim stress showed an increased ulcer index, volume of gastric content, free and total acidity, and MDA level; and a decreased total carbohydrate to total protein ratio, ascorbic acid, SOD and CAT level. Rats treated with WS and subjected to stress showed a reversal of the changes observed in rats subjected to stress without WS treatment. The effect of WS (100 mg/kg) was comparable to ranitidine (30 mg/kg, P.O.).

Raghuveer and coworkers[9] examined the effect of ethanol extract of Withania somnifera root (WS) on ethanol-induced ulceration in rats. Adult male albino rats treated with WS (250 and 500 mg/kg, P.O.) followed by ethanol (80%, 1 ml/kg, P.O.) showed a significant reduction in ulcer incidence and ulcer index compared to rats treated with ethanol without WS.

Nair and coworkers[10] reported that a polyherbal formulation (NR-ANX-C) containing an aqueous extract of Withania somnifera root was more effective than the standard drug ranitidine against aspirin or pyloric ligature-induced gastric ulceration in rats.

References

1   H. Pylori and Peptic ulcers. NIH Publication No 10-4225, National Digestive Diseases Information Clearinghouse (NDDIC), Bethesda, MD, 2010.

2   NSAIDs and peptic ulcers. National Digestive Diseases Information Clearinghouse, Bethesda, MD (2010). NIH Publication No. 10-4664

3   Peter Malfertheiner, Francis K L Chan, Kenneth E L McColl. Peptic ulcer disease. The Lancet (2009) 374: 1449-1461.

4   N. Singh, R. Nath, A. Lata, S. P. Singh, R. P. Kohli and K. P. Bhargava. Withania somnifera (Ashwagandha), a rejuvenating herbal drug which enhances survival during stress (an adaptogen). International Journal of Crude Drug Research (1982) 20 (1): 29-35.

5   Salil K. Bhattacharya, Raj K. Goel, Ravinder Kaur and Shibnath Ghosal. Anti-stress activity of sitoindosides VII and VIII, new acylsterylglucosides from Withania somnifera. Phytotherapy Research (1987) 1 (1): 32-37.

6   B. Singh, A. K. Saxena, B. K. Chandan, D. K. Gupta, K. K. Bhutani and K. K. Anand. Adaptogenic activity of a novel, Withanolide-free aqueous fraction from the roots of Withania somnifera Dun. Phytotherapy Research (2001) 15: 311-318.

7   S. K. Bhattacharya, A. V. Muruganandam. Adaptogenic activity of Withania somnifera: an experimental study using a rat model of chronic stress. Pharmacology, Biochemistry and Behavior (2003) 75: 547-555.

8   Bhatnagar M, Jain C P and Sisodia S S. Anti-ulcer activity of Withania somnifera in stress plus pyloric ligation induced gastric ulcer in rats. Journal of Cell and Tissue Research (2005) 5 (1): 287-292.

9   Raghuveer B, Chakravarthy K and Umamaheswara Raju S. Evaluation of preventive effect of Withania somnifera root extract against ethanol induced ulcers in rats. International Journal of Bioassays (2013) 2 (6): 938-941.

10 Vinod Nair, Albina Arjuman, H. N. Gopalakrishna, P. Dorababu, Mirshad P. V, Divya Bhargavan & Dipsanker Chatterji. Evaluation of the anti-ulcer activity of NR-ANX-C (a polyherbal formulation) in aspirin & pyloric ligature induced gastric ulcers in albino rats. Indian J Med Res (2010) 132: 218-232.

16 – Immunomodulatory Activity

16.1 – Introduction

Immunity is the general ability of the body to resist infection or disease[1]. The immune system can distinguish between self (proteins and other molecules made by one's body) and other (proteins and other molecules not made by one's body). There are two major components of the immune system: innate immunity and adaptive immunity. Innate immunity, also called natural immunity, is inborn. It provides an immediate, non-specific first line of defense against invading toxins and pathogens. Adaptive immunity, also called acquired immunity, develops only after exposure to a pathogen. It is highly specific to the pathogen and improves with repeated exposure.

The immune system consists of a complex network of cells, tissues, organs and molecules that work together. Natural or synthetic substances that stimulate, suppress or regulate the innate and adaptive arms of the immune system are known as immunomodulators[2]. A number of studies have examined the immunomodulatory effects of Withania somnifera and the results are summarized below.

16.2 – Summary of Results

Ghosal and coworkers[3] isolated two glycowithanolides (sitoindosides IX and X) from Withania somnifera and tested their immunomodulatory effect in Swiss mice. Mice treated with compound IX or X (100-400 µg) produced mobilization and activation of peritoneal macrophages, phagocytosis, and enhanced activity of lysosomal enzymes secreted by the activated macrophages.

Ziauddin and coworkers[4] investigated the immunomodulatory effects of Withania somnifera (WS) in mice using the model of myelo- and immuno-suppression drugs. Albino mice were sensitized with a thymus-dependent antigen and treated with cyclophosphamide (3 mg/kg/day, P.O.), prednisolone (5 mg/kg/day, P.O.), azathioprin (3 mg/kg/day, P.O.), cyclophosphamide+WS (100 mg/

kg/day, P.O.), prednisolone+WS (100 mg/kg/day, P.O.) or azathio-prin+WS (100 mg/kg/day, P.O.) for 15 days. Some mice from each group were sacrificed on day 16 and blood was collected for analysis. The rest were reimmunized with the same antigen. On day 22, these mice were sacrificed and blood was collected for analysis. Mice treated with cyclophosphamide, prednisolone or azathioprin and sacrificed on day 16 showed a decrease in hemoglobin, RBC count, platelet count and white blood cell count compared to controls. Mice treated with WS along with cyclophosphamide, prednisolone or azathioprin and sacrificed on day 16 showed a mitigation of the changes induced by the drugs. Mice sacrificed on day 21 showed a similar response. The authors concluded that "The use of Ashwagandha as an immunomodulator to counteract the undesirable effects of myelosuppressive drugs and also for developing and improving protective immunity even in normal individuals may be possible in the future".

Dhuley[5] examined the effect of Withania somnifera (WS) on the functions of macrophages in mice treated with the carcinogen ochratoxin A (OTA). Mice treated with OTA showed decreased macrophage chemotactic activity as well as reduced production of interleukin-1 and tumor necrosis factor-α. Treatment with WS attenuated the changes induced by OTA.

Davis and Kuttan[6] studied the immunological potential of a methanol (70%) extract of Withania somnifera roots (WS) in mice treated with a non-lethal dose of cyclophosphamide (CTX). Female Swiss albino mice treated with CTX (25 mg/kg/day) for 10 days showed a lower WBC count on the 12th day compared to CTX (25 mg/kg)+WS (20 mg/day)-treated mice. Also, the CTX+WS treated group showed more bone marrow cellularity and α-esterase positive cells in the bone marrow compared to the CTX group. In a subsequent investigation, Davis and Kuttan[7] examined the effect of a Withania somnifera root extract on cyclophosphamide-treated mice. Treatment of cyclophosphamide-treated Balb/c mice with WS increased the levels of IFN-γ, IL-2 and GM-CSF. Irradiated mice treated with bone marrow cells extracted from WS-treated mice showed increased spleen nodular colonies compared to irradiated mice treated with bone marrow cells from mice not treated with WS. In another investigation, Davis and Kuttan[8] observed that treating Balb/c mice with a methanol (70%) extract of Withania somnifera roots (20 mg, i.p.) for 5 days showed an increase in total WBC count, bone marrow cells and α-esterase positive cells, as well as an increase in thymus and spleen size and weight compared to controls. Mice immunized with sheep red blood cells (SRBC) and treated with the extract showed an increased antibody titre and number of plaque-forming cells compared to immunized mice not treated with the extract. The extract inhibited the delayed type hypersensitivity response in mice and enhanced the phagocytic activity of peritoneal macrophages.

Iuvone and coworkers[9] studied the effect of a methanol extract of Withania somnifera roots (WS) on the production of NO in J774 macrophages. J774 macrophage cells treated with WS (1-256 μg/ml) showed a concentration-dependent increase in nitrite levels compared to macrophages not treated with WS. The production of nitrite in WS (256 μg/ml)-treated cells was inhibited by L-NAME (NO synthase inhibitor) or TLCK (inhibitor of NF-κB activation). Adding dexamethasone (inhibitor of protein synthesis) to cells before adding WS also inhibited nitrite production. However, adding dexamethasone 12 hours after adding WS showed no effect on nitrite production. An immunoblotting analysis of iNOS protein expression in cells incubated with WS showed increased iNOS protein expression compared to cells not treated with WS. The authors concluded that "Our results show for the first time that WS stimulates macrophage-derived NO production, and is able to up-regulate iNOS expression through NF-κB transactivation in murine macrophages".

Gautam and coworkers[10] investigated the immunomodulatory effect of an aqueous extract of Withania somnifera roots (WS) in mice immunized with a DPT (Diphtheria, Pertussis, Tetanus) vaccine. Swiss albino mice immunized with the vaccine and treated with WS (100 mg/kg/day) for 15 days showed increased serum antibody titers to B. pertussis compared to mice immunized with the vaccine and not treated with WS. The mice then received an intracerebral challenge with live B. pertussis cells. On day 28 of the study, immunized WS-treated mice showed increased pertussis antibody titers and reduced morbidity and mortality compared to immunized mice not treated with WS. The authors concluded that the "Present study indicates application of [WS] as potential immunopotentiating agent [with] possible applications in immunochemical industry".

Bani and coworkers[11] demonstrated that an aqueous extract of Withania somnifera root (WSE) selectively upregulated Th1-type cytokines in immunized mice. Immunized (SRBC) Balb/c mice treated with WSE for 7 days and challenged with SRBC on the 6th day showed increased IFN-γ and IL-2 (Th1 cytokines) in the blood and no significant change in IL-4 (Th-2 cytokine) compared to immunized and challenged mice not treated with WSE. A similar experiment with levamisole (positive control) instead of WSE showed an increase in IFN-γ, IL-2 and IL-4. Mice treated with cyclosporin two days before immunization showed decreased blood levels of CD4+ and CD8+ 7 days after immunization compared to immunized mice not pretreated with cyclosporin. Immunized mice pretreated with cyclosporin and treated with WSE for 7 days showed attenuation of the CD4+ and CD8+ changes induced by cyclosporin. The authors concluded that "This study indicates the selective Th1 up-regulating effect of extract and suggests its use for selective Th1/Th2 modulation".

Khan and coworkers[12] reported that a standardized aqueous extract of Withania somnifera roots mitigated chronic stress-induced depletion of T cells and Th-1 type cytokines in BALB/c mice.

Gupta and coworkers[13] reported that for Wistar albino rats immunized and challenged by SRBC, orally administering Ashwagandha churna (powder preparation) increased neutrophile adhesion and the delayed-type hypersensitivity response.

Rasool and Varalakshmi[14] examined the immunomodulatory effects of an aqueous suspension of Withania somnifera root powder in vivo and in vitro. Withania somnifera exhibited inhibitory activity towards the complement system, mitogen-induced lymphocyte proliferation and the delayed-type hypersensitivity reaction. Withania somnifera (1000 mg/kg) did not show a significant effect on the humoral immune response in rats.

Malik and coworkers[15] investigated the immunomodulatory activity of a standardized alcohol-water (1:1) extract of Withania somnifera roots (AGB) in SRBC-immunized mice. BALB/c mice were treated with saline (control) or AGB (10, 30 or 100 mg/kg/day, P.O.) for 9 days and immunized by injecting SRBC on the 9th day. Treatment with saline or AGB was continued till day 15. The following observations were made in the AGB group compared to the control group:

- splenocytes showed an increased population of T cells upon stimulation with Con A and a similar effect on B cells upon stimulation with LPS

- splenocytes showed increased production of Th1 cytokines (IFN-γ and IL-2) and a decrease in the Th2 cytokine IL-4 upon stimulation with Con A

- peritoneal macrophages showed increased production of IL-12, TNF-α and NO, but no change in IL-10

The following observations were made in mice treated with AGB for 15 days that were immunized and challenged on days 9 and 15 respectively:

- significant DTH response
- increased serum IgM titer and IgG antibodies

The authors concluded that "AGB is a potent immunostimulatory agent, which can be therapeutically used in enhancing the immune response in diseases like tuberculosis, cancer, leishmaniasis, leprosy and AIDS".

Yamada and coworkers[16] reported that Withania somnifera increased immunoglobulin production in rat spleen lymphocytes.

Kanyaiya and coworkers[17] studied the immunomodulatory potential of an aqueous extract of Withania somnifera (WS) in mice. Swiss albino mice were treated with a normal synthetic diet+milk (control), a normal synthetic diet containing 0.3% WS (group A) or a normal synthetic diet containing 0.3% WS+milk (group B) for 28 days. Peritoneal macrophages from groups A and B showed increased phagocytic activity compared to the control group. Serum from groups A and B showed increased IgG compared to the control group.

Kumari and coworkers[18] demonstrated the immunomodulatory effects of a methanol (70%) extract of Withania somnifera roots (WSE) in vitro and in vivo. Treatment of lymphocytes isolated from healthy dog blood with WSE increased lymphocyte proliferation compared to controls. Treatment of dexamethasone-induced immunocompromised mice with WSE improved primary and secondary antibody titers compared to controls.

Naik and coworkers[19] demonstrated the immunomodulatory activity of a Withania somnifera extract using various animal models: cyclophosphamide-induced immunosuppression, phagocytosis by carbon clearance and delayed type hypersensitivity.

Verma and coworkers[20] showed that an ethanol whole plant extract of Withania somnifera enhanced both humoral and cell-mediated immune responses in mice.

References

1   Lansing M Prescott, John P Harley, Donald A Klein. Microbiology, Fifth Edition. McGraw Hill, New York, 2005.

2   Dinesh Kumar, Vikrant Arya, Ranjeet Kaur, Zulfiqar Ali Bhat, Vivek Kumar Gupta, Vijender Kumar. A review of immunomodulators in the Indian traditional health care system. Journal of Microbiology, Immunology and Infection (2012) 45: 165-184.

3   Shibnath Ghosal, Jawahar Lal, Radheyshyam Srivastava, Salil K. Bhattacharya, Sachidananda N. Upadhyay, Arun K. Jaiswal, Utpala Chattopadhyay. Immunomodulatory and CNS effects of sitoindosides IX and X, two new glycowithanolides from Withania somnifera. Phytotherapy Research (1989) 3(5): 201-206.

4   Mohammed Ziauddin, Neeta Phansalkar, Pralhad Patki, Sham Diwanay, Bhusan Patwardhan. Studies on the immunomodulatory effects of Ashwagandha. Journal of Ethnopharmacology (1996) 50: 69-76.

5   J N Dhuley. Effect of some Indian herbs on macrophage functions in ochratoxin A treated mice. Journal of Ethnopharmacology (1997) 58(1): 15-20.

6   Leemol Davis, Girija Kuttan. Suppressive effect of cyclophosphamide-induced toxicity by Withania somnifera extract in mice. Journal of Ethnopharmacology (1998) 62: 209-214.

7   Leemol Davis, Girija Kuttan. Effect of Withania somnifera on cytokine production in normal and cyclophosphamide treated mice. Immunopharmacol Immunotoxicol (1999) 21(4): 695-703.

8   Leemol Davis, Girija Kuttan. Immunomodulatory activity of Withania somnifera. Journal of Ethnopharmacology (2000) 71: 193-200.

9   Teresa Iuvone, Giuseppe Esposito, Francesco Capasso, Angelo A. Izzo. Induction of nitric oxide synthase expression by Withania somnifera in macrophages. Life Sciences (2003) 72: 1617-1625.

10 M. Gautam, S. S. Diwanny, S. Gairola, Y. S. Shinde, S. S. Jadhav, B. K. Patwardhan. Immune response modulation to DPT vaccine by aqueous extract of Withania somnifera in experimental system. International Immunopharmacology (2004) 4: 841-849.

11 Sarang Bani, Manish Gautam, Fayaz Ahmad Sheikh, Beenish Khan, Narender Kumar Satti, Krishan Avtar Suri, Ghulam Nabi Qazi, Bhushan Patwardhan. Selective Th1 up-regulating activity of Withania somnifera aqueous extract in an experimental system using flow cytometry. Journal of Ethnopharmacology (2006) 107: 107-115.

12 Benish Khan, Sheikh Fayaz Ahmad, Sarang Bani, Anpurna Kaul, K. A. Suri, N. K. Satti, M. Athar, G. N. Qazi. Augmentation and proliferation of T lymphocytes and Th-1 cytokines by Withania somnifera in stressed mice. International Immunopharmacology (2006) 6: 1394-1403.

13 M. Suresh Gupta, H. N. Shivaprasad, M. D. Kharya and A.C. Rana. Immunomodulatory activity of Ayurvedic formulation "Ashwagandha Churna". Pharmaceutical Biology (2006) 44 (4): 263-265.

14 M. Rasool, P.Varalakshmi. Immunomodulatory role of Withania somnifera root powder on experimental induced inflammation: An in vivo and in Vitro study. Vascular Pharmacology (2006) 44: 406-410.

15 Fayaz Malik, Jaswant Singh, Anamika Khajuria, Krishan A. Suri, Naresh K. Satti, Surjeet Singh, Maharaj K. Kaul, Arun Kumar, Aruna Bhatia, Ghulam N. Qazi. A standardized root extract of Withania somnifera and its major

constituent withanolide-A elicit humoral and cell-mediated immune responses by upregulation of Th1-dominant polarization in BALB/c mice. Life Sciences (2007) 80: 1525-1538.

16 Koji Yamada, Pham Hung, Tae Kyu Park, Pyo Jam Park, Beong Ou Lim. A comparison of the immunostimulatory effects of the medicinal herbs Echinacea, Ashwagandha and Brahmi. Journal of Ethnopharmacology (2011) 137: 231-235.

17 Moharkar Kanyaiya, Sawale Pravin Digambar, Sumit Arora, Suman Kapila & R. R. B. Singh. In vivo, effect of herb (Withania somnifera) on immunomodulatory and antioxidative potential of milk in mice. Food and Agricultural Immunology (2014) 25(3): 443-452.

18 Priyambada Kumari, Shanker K. Singh, Umesh Dimri, Meena Kataria, Sushma Ahlawat. Immunostimulatory activities of Withania somnifera root extract in dexamethasone induced immunocompromised mice and in vitro model. Asian Journal of Complementary and Alternative Medicine (2014) 2(2): 6-10.

19 Suresh R. Naik, Chetan Gavankar and Vishnu N. Thakare. Immunomodulatory activity of Withania somnifera and Curcuma longa in animal models: Modulation of cytokines functioning. Pharmacologia (2015) 6(5): 168-177.

20 Satish K. Verma, Asima Shaban, Reena Purohit, Madhvi L. Chimata, Geeta Rai and Om Prakash Verma. Immunomodulatory activity of Withania somnifera (L). Journal of Chemical and Pharmaceutical Research (2012) 4 (1): 559-561.

17 – Anti-inflammatory Activity

17.1 – Introduction

Inflammation is the body's defense response to harmful stimuli such as pathogens, damaged cells, toxic chemicals or physical injury. Four cardinal signs of inflammation are redness, heat, swelling and pain. The inflammatory response involves dilation of blood vessels, increased blood flow, increased vascular permeability, exudation of fluids, and mediator release, among other activities[1]. This helps to neutralize harmful stimuli and initiate the healing process[2]. Inflammation can be acute or chronic. Acute inflammation is a short time response and usually results in healing. Chronic inflammation persists for a long time, attacks the body and contributes to the development of a variety of diseases[3]. A number of studies have been conducted on the anti-inflammatory activity of Withania somnifera and the results are summarized below.

17.2 – Summary of Results

Anbalagan and Sadique[4] reported the anti-inflammatory activity of Withania Somnifera roots (WS) on adjuvant-induced inflammation in rats. Rats were treated with WS (1 g/kg, P.O.) one hour before the induction of inflammation by Freund's complete adjuvant (FCA). WS treatment was continued for 3 days, and the inflammation induced by FCA was reduced. Also, WS changed the concentration of many serum proteins produced during the acute phase of inflammation. In another study, Anbalagan and Sadique[5] found that Withania somnifera caused a dose-dependent suppression of alpha-2 macroglobulin (an indicator for anti-inflammatory drugs) and enhancement of total proteins in the serum of rats given a subplantar injection of carrageenan suspension.

Begum and Sadique[6] examined the effect of Withania Somnifera (WS) on glycosaminoglycan synthesis in carrageenan-induced air pouch granuloma. Air pouch granuloma was induced by subcutaneously injecting carrageenan (2%, 4 ml) on the dorsum of male

Wistar albino rats which had been injected (S.C.) with 6 ml of air one day before. Rats bearing 7-day-old granulomas were treated with saline (control), WS (1000 mg/kg, P.O.), hydrocortisone (15 mg/kg, P.O.) or phenylbutazone (100 mg/kg, P.O.) twice daily from day 7 to 9. On the 9th day, the animals were injected with $Na_2^{35}SO_4$ (50 μCi, i.p).

The animals were sacrificed on the 10th day. The WS and hydrocortisone groups showed a 55% and 46% decrease, respectively, in glycosaminoglycan content in granulation tissue compared to controls. Also, the WS and hydrocortisone groups showed a significant decrease in monosulfated and highly sulfated glycosaminoglycans as well as a decrease in the incorporation of labeled sulfate into glycosaminoglycans. The phenylbutazone group did not show much effect. WS was found to effect uncoupling of oxidative phosphorylation by reducing the ratio of ADP/O. Also, WS increased Mg^{2+}-dependent ATPase enzyme activity and decreased succinate dehydrogenase activity in the mitochondria of the granulation tissue. Neither hydrocortisone or phenylbutazone showed such effects. The authors suggested that "W. somnifera is able to inhibit glycosaminoglycan biosynthesis mainly through the inhibition of ATP biogenesis".

In another study, Begum and Sadique[7] investigated the effect of Withania somnifera on Freund's complete adjuvant-induced arthritis in rats. Treatment of arthritic rats with WS (1000 mg/kg/day, P.O.) for 15 days caused a reduction in paw swelling and bony degenerative changes. WS was more effective than hydrocortisone (15 mg/kg).

Al-Hindawi and coworkers[8] reported that an ethanol (80%) extract of Withania somnifera suppressed carrageenan-induced paw edema in albino Wistar rats. The effect of 76.4 mg/kg WS (1/10 LD_{50}) was comparable to 200 mg/kg of acetylsalicylic acid. In another investigation, Al-Hindawi and coworkers[9] found that various fractions of a methanol (70%) extract of Withania somnifera aerial parts inhibited granuloma formation induced by subcutaneously implanted cotton pellets in albino Wistar rats.

Sahni and Srivastava[10] demonstrated the anti-inflammatory activity of an aqueous extract of Withania somnifera roots (WS) on carrageenan-induced inflammation in rats. Norwegian inbred albino rats were treated with saline or WS (500, 750 or 1000 mg/kg, P.O.) and injected with carrageenan. WS-treated rats showed significantly reduced paw edema (69%) compared to the saline group. The anti-inflammatory activity was possibly due to WS inhibiting release of the inflammation mediators histamine, 5-HT and prostaglandins.

Jayaprakasam and Nair[11] isolated several compounds listed below from a Withania somnifera leaf extract and tested their ability to inhibit cyclooxygenase-2 (COX-2) enzyme activity. All compounds except 9 showed selective COX-2 inhibition.

1	Physagulin D (1→6)-β-D-glucopyranosyl(1→4)-β-D-glucopyranoside
2	27-O-β-D-glucopyranosyl physagulin D
3	27-O-β-D-glucopyranosyl viscosalactone B
4	4,16-dihyroxy-5β,6β-epoxyphysagulin D
5	4-(1-hydroxy-2,2-dimethylcyclo-propanone)-2,3-dihydrowithaferin A
6	Withaferin A
7	2,3-dihydrowithaferin A
8	Viscosalactone B
9	27-desoxy-24,25-dihydrowithaferin A
10	Sitoindoside IX
11	Physagulin D
12	Withanoside IV

Table 17.1: Compounds isolated from a Withania somnifera leaf extract

Rasol and Varalakshmi[12] demonstrated the anti-inflammatory activity of Withania somnifera roots (WS) in arthritic rats. 72 hours after injection with complete Freund's adjuvant (CFA) in the right hind paw, Albino Wistar rats showed a 135% increase in footpad thickness. Rats treated with WS 1 hour before CFA injection and then treated with WS for 5 days showed only a 62.5% increase in footpad thickness. Another investigation[13] made the following observations 19 days after intradermal injection with CFA compared to controls:

- increased plasma and spleen LPO
- diminished spleen antioxidants
- increased plasma protein-bound carbohydrates and spleen protein-bound carbohydrates
- decreased bone collagen and increased urinary excretions

Rats injected with CFA and after 11 days treated with WS (1000 mg/kg/day, P.O.) for 8 days showed a reversal of the changes observed in arthritic rats not treated with WS.

In vitro studies by Singh and coworkers[14] found that an ethanol (95%) extract of Withania somnifera roots (WS) suppressed the production of pro-inflammatory molecules in peripheral blood mononuclear cells (PBMCs) from normal human subjects and rheumatoid arthritis (RA) patients. WS treatment of normal PBMCs suppressed spontaneous production of TNF-α, IL-1β and IL-6 but showed no effect on IL-12p40. WS treatment of normal PBMCs suppressed LPS-induced production of TNF-α, IL-1β and IL-12p40 but showed no effect on IL-6. WS treatment of RA PBMCs suppressed spontaneous production of all four cytokines but only suppressed LPS-induced production of TNF-α, IL-1β and IL-12p40, with no effect on IL-6. WS treatment of normal and RA PBMCs inhibited LPS-induced phosphorylation of IκBα and nuclear translocation of NF-κB and AP-1. WS inhibited LPS-induced production of nitric oxide in the mouse macrophage cell line RAW 264.7.

Sabina and coworkers[15] examined the effect of Withaferin A on monosodium urate (MSU)-induced inflammation in mice, an experimental model for gouty arthritis. Swiss albino mice injected with MSU (4 mg/0.2 ml) intradermally into the right footpad showed the following changes compared to controls:

- increased paw volume
- increased serum, liver and spleen lysosomal enzymes
- increased plasma, liver and spleen LPO and TNF-α
- decreased liver and spleen enzymatic antioxidants

WA (30 mg/kg/day, i.p.) or indomethacin (3 mg/kg/day, i.p.) treatment an hour before MSU injection and subsequently for 3 days attenuated the changes induced by MSU. The effect of WA was comparable to indomethacin. The authors concluded that "The present findings clearly indicated that Withaferin A exerted a strong anti-inflammatory effect against gouty arthritis".

Ganesan and coworkers[16] reported that an ethanol-water (1:3) extract of Withania somnifera inhibited the degradation of collagen by Clostridium histolyticcum collagenase (Chc). Chc belongs to the M-31 metalloproteinase family. It is capable of hydrolyzing collagens under physiological conditions. The mechanism of its action has been considered to be similar to mammalian matrix metalloproteinases. Bovine achilles tendons (BAT) treated with various amounts of the extract and incubated with Chc showed a dose-dependent decrease in the degradation of collagen compared to BAT incubated with Chc in the absence of the extract.

The anti-inflammatory activity of a hydro-alcoholic (3:7) extract of Withania somnifera (WS) was examined by Sharma and Sharma[17]. The human red blood cell membrane stabilization method and albumin denaturation assay were used. A suspension of human red blood cells was incubated with or without WS. WS inhibited membrane lyses in a concentration-dependent manner. Bovine serum albumin was incubated with or without WS. WS inhibited protein denaturation in a dose-dependent manner.

Srinivasulu[18] reported that an aqueous extract of Withania somnifera root inhibited the production of pro-inflammatory cytokines (TNF-α, IL-1) as well as NO in J774 murine macrophage cells stimulated by LPS.

Amabeoku and coworkers[19] reported that an aqueous extract of Withania somnifera leaves reduced paw edema in rats induced by injecting carrageenan into the subplantar surface of the right hind paw.

Gupta and Singh[20] evaluated the anti-inflammatory effect of Withania somnifera root extract (WS) on collagen-induced arthritis in rats. Bovine tracheal cartilage type II (CII) was emulsified with Freund's adjuvant incomplete (IFA). Albino female Wistar rats were intradermally injected with the CII/IFA emulsion at several sites on the back and reimmunized seven days later. Rats were then observed for 45 days for the development and progression of arthritis. The following changes were observed on the 45th day compared to controls: swelling, redness, deformity and ankylosis in the hind paw and ankle joints, arthritic pain, diminished rotarod activity, increased paw thickness and ankle size, decreased body weight, increased arthritic score, reduction in sciatic function index, bone erosion and joint space narrowing in the ankle joint. Rats treated with WS (600 mg/kg/day, P.O.) on days 20-45 showed a reversal of these changes. The authors concluded that "W. somnifera treatment could be a potential therapeutic strategy for the treatment of RA".

Balkrishna and coworkers[21] examined the effect of Ashwashila (ASHW) on rheumatoid arthritis symptoms. ASHW is a herbomineral formulation containing equal amounts of an aqueous extract of Ashwagandha and Shilajit. Rheumatoid arthritis was induced in Balb/c mice by injecting a collagen antibody cocktail and lipopolysaccharide (i.p.). Arthritic mice treated with the vehicle (0.25% Na-CMC, P.O.) every day for two weeks showed the following changes compared to controls (normal Balb/c mice treated with PBS+0.25% Na-CMC for two weeks):

- reduced food and water consumption and body weight
- increased pedal edema and increased paw and ankle arthritic scores
- increased radiological and histological lesion scores in the ankle joint, knee joint and articular cartilage

Arthritic mice treated with ASHW (353 mg/kg/day, P.O.) for two weeks reversed these changes except for the reduced food and water consumption. The antiarthritic mechanism of ASHW was explored by in vitro studies. Human monocyte THP-1 cells stimulated with LPS showed upregulation of pro-inflammatory cytokines such as IL-1β, IL-6 and INF-α and the upstream regulatory protein NF-κB. Treatment with ASHW reduced these changes in a dose-dependent manner. The authors concluded that "Ashwashila can be a potential candidate for treating rheumatoid arthritis, as a standalone or companion therapy".

Khan and coworkers[22] examined the antiarthritic activity of an aqueous extract of Withania somnifera root (WSAq) in collagen-induced arthritic (CIA) rats. Arthritis was induced in male Wistar albino rats by injecting an emulsion of bovine type II collagen (S.C.) and complete Freund's adjuvant at the base of the tail. CIA rats were treated with saline or WSAq (300 mg/kg/day, P.O.) for 20 days. Normal male Wistar albino rats treated with saline served as controls. CIA rats treated with saline showed increased paw and ankle thickness, increased levels of pro-inflammatory cytokines (TNF-α, IL-1β, IL-6), increased transcription factor NF-κB, decreased IL-10, increased MMP-8, increased iNOS mRNA, increased activity of CAT and GPx, decreased SOD activity, and histopathological changes in paw joints compared to controls. CIA rats treated with WSAq showed a reversal of the changes observed in CIA rats. The effect of WSAq was comparable to methotrexate (0.25 mg/kg, i.p.). The authors concluded that "the use of WSAq300 may be a valuable supplement which can improve human arthritis".

Giri[23] conducted a comparative study of the anti-inflammatory activities of an ethanol extract of Withania somnifera (WS) and hydrocortisone in rats. In an acute study, Wistar albino rats treated with WS (12 or 25 mg/kg, P.O.) or hydrocortisone (40 mg/kg, S.C.) followed by subplantar injection of carrageenan to the right hind paw showed less paw edema compared to rats injected with carrageenan without any pretreatment. In a chronic study, rats were treated with WS (25 mg/kg, P.O.) or hydrocortisone (40 mg/kg, S.C.) followed by subplantar injection of complete Freund's adjuvant and further treatment with WS or hydrocortisone for 12 days. The WS and hydrocortisone groups showed less paw edema compared to rats injected with carrageenan without any pre/post treatment. The effect of WS was comparable to hydrocortisone.

Kulkarni and coworkers[24] conducted a double-blind, placebo-controlled cross-over study to evaluate the effectiveness of a herbomineral formulation in the treatment of osteoarthritis. Each capsule of the formulation contained Withania somnifera (450 mg), Boswellia (100 mg), Curcuma longa (50 mg) and a zinc complex (50 mg). 42 patients with osteoarthritis were randomized to receive the formulation (2 capsules/day) or placebo for three months. After a washout period of 15 days, the subjects were transferred to the other treatment for 3 months. Pain and disability scores were evaluated weekly. Erythrocyte sedimentation rate (ESR) and radiological studies were done monthly. The herbomineral formulation treatment reduced the severity of pain and disability scores. No significant changes in ESR or radiological appearance were observed.

Ramakanth and coworkers[25] conducted a randomized, double-blind, placebo-controlled study to evaluate the efficacy and tolerability of a standardized extract of Withania somnifera (roots and leaves) in patients with knee joint pain and discomfort. 60 patients with knee joint pain and discomfort were randomized into 3 groups. The first and the second groups were treated with 250 mg and 125 mg of the extract, respectively, twice a day for 4 weeks. The third group received a placebo. Paracetamol was given as and when needed. At the end of 12 weeks, the extract-treated groups showed a reduction in the Modified Western Ontario and McMaster University Osteoarthritis Index (mWOMAC), Knee Swelling Index, and VAS scores for pain, stiffness and disability compared to baseline and the placebo group. The 250 mg dose was more effective than the 125 mg dose. The extract-treated groups consumed less paracetamol than the placebo group, and the treatment was well tolerated without serious side effects.

Mariappan and coworkers[26] reported that treating RA patients with Withania somnifera in honey (2 or 4 g/day) for 49 days reduced RA symptoms and inflammatory parameters, and improved blood hemoglobin, kidney and liver functions.

References

1   P. Padmanabhan and S. N. Jangle. Evaluation of in vitro anti-inflammatory activity of herbal preparation, a combination of four medicinal plants. International Journal of Basic and Applied Medical Sciences (2012) 2(1): 109-116.

2   Juan Jesus Carrero and Peter Stenvinkel. Persistent inflammation as a catalyst for risk factors in chronic kidney disease: a hypothesis proposal. Clin J Am Soc Nephrol (2009) 4: S49-S55.

3   Linlin Chen, Huidan Deng, Hengmin Cui, Jing Fang, Zhicai Zuo, Junliang Deng, Yinglum Li, Xun Wang and Ling Zhao. Inflammatory responses and inflammation associated diseases in organs. Oncotarget (2018) 9 (6): 7204-7218.

4   K. Anbalagan and J. Sadique. Influence of an Indian medicine (Ashwagandha) on acute phase reactants in inflammation. Indian J. of Experimental Biology (1981) 19: 245-249.

5   K. Anbalagan and J. Sadique. Withania somnifera (Ashwagandha), a rejuvenating herbal drug which controls alpha-2-macroglobulin synthesis during inflammation. Int. J. Crude Drug Res (1985) 23 (4): 177-183.

6   V. H. Begum and J. Sadique. Effect of Withania somnifera on glycosaminoglycan synthesis in carrageenan induced air pouch granuloma. Biochem Med Metab Biol (1987) 38 (3): 272-277.

7   V. H. Begum and J Sadique. Long term effect of herbal drug Withania somnifera on adjuvant induced arthritis in rats. Indian J Exp Biol (1988) 26: 877-882.

8   Muhaned K. Al-Hindawi, Ihsan H. S. Al-Deen, May H.A. Nabi and Mudafar A. Ismail. Antiinflammatory activity of some Iraqi plants using intact rats. Journal of Ethnopharmacology (1989) 26: 163-168.

9   Muhaned K. Al-Hindawi, Saadia H. Al-Khafaji and May H. Abdul-Nabi. Anti-granuloma activity of Iraqi Withania somnifera. Journal of Ehnopharmacology (1992) 37: 113-116.

10 Y. P. Sahni, D. N. Srivastava. Anti-inflammatory activity of Withania somnifera: possible mode of action. J. Appl. Anim Res (1993) 3: 129-136.

11 Bolleddula Jayaprakasam and Muraleedharan G. Nair. Cyclooxygenase-2 enzyme inhibitory withanolides from Withania somnifera leaves. Tetrahedron (2003) 59: 841-849.

12 M. Rasool, P. Varalakshmi. Immunomodulatory role of Withania somnifera root powder on experimental induced inflammation: an in vivo and in vitro study. Vacular Pharmacology (2006) 44: 406-410.

13 M. Rasool, P. Varalakshmi. Protective effect of Withania somnifera root powder in relation to lipid peroxidation, antioxidant status, glycoproteins and bone collagen on adjuvant-induced arthritis in rats. Fundamental & Clinical Pharmacology (2007) 21: 157-164.

14 Divya Singh, Amita Aggarwal, Rakesh Maurya and Sita Naik. Withania somnifera inhibits NF-κB and AP-1 transcription factors in human peripheral blood and synovial fluid mononuclear cells. Phytother. Res (2007) 21: 905-913.

15 Evan Prince Sabina, Sonal Chandel and Mahaboob Khan Rasool. Inhibition of monosodium urate crystal-induced inflammation by Withaferin A. J Pharm Pharmaceut Sci (2008) 11(4): 46-55.

16 Krishnamoorthy Ganesan, Praveen Kumar Sehgal, Asit Baran Mandal, Sadulla Sayeed. Protective effect of Withania somnifera and Cardiospermum

halicacabum extracts against collagenolytic degradation of collagen. Appl
Biochem Biotechnol (2011) 165: 1075-1091.

17 Lalit Sharma and Arun Sharma. In vitro antioxidant, anti-inflammatory, and
antimicrobial activity of hydro-alcoholic extract of roots of Withania
somnifera. Journal of Chemical and Pharmaceutical Research (2014) 6
(7):178-182.

18 Amara Srinivasulu. Anti-inflammatory effects of aqueous extract of Withania
somnifera on LPS- stimulated pro-inflammatory mediators in J774 murine
macrophages. International Journal of Scientific Research (2014) 3 (1): 15-17.

19 George Jimboyeka Amabeoku, Oluchi Nneka Mbamalu, Munira Ismail,
Nabeel Dudhia, Nadeem Noordien, Zukiswa Mabuya and Oatlhostse
Kakutsi. Evaluation of the anti-inflammatory and sedative effects of leaf
aqueous extract of Withania somnifera(L.) Dunal (Solanaceae) in rats and
mice. Journal of Pharmacy and Pharmacology (2015) 3: 469-478.

20 Apurva Gupta & Surendra Singh. Evaluation of anti-inflammatory effect of
Withania somnifera root on collagen-induced arthritis in rats. Pharmaceutical
Biology (2014) 52 (3): 308-320.

21 Acharya Balkrishna, Sachin Shridhar Sakat, Kheemraj Joshi, Sandeep
Paudel, Deepika Joshi, Kamal Joshi, Ravikant Ranjan, Abhishek Gupta,
Kunal Bhattacharya & Anurag Varshney. Herbo-mineral formulation
Ashwashila attenuates rheumatoid arthritis symptoms in collagen- antibody-
induced arthritis (CAIA) mice model. Scientific Reports (2019) 9: 8025.

22 Mahmood Ahmad Khan, Rafat Sultana Ahmed, Nilesh Chandra, Vinod
Kumar Arora and Athar Ali. In vivo, extract from Withania somnifera root
ameliorates arthritis via regulation of key immune mediators of inflammation
in experimental model of arthritis. Anti-Inflammatory & Anti-Allergy Agents
in Medicinal Chemistry (2019) 18: 55-70.

23 Kiran R Giri. Comparative study of anti-inflammatory activity of Withania
somnifera (Ashwagandha) with hydrocortisone in experimental animals
(Albino rats). Journal of Medicinal Plant Studies (2016) 4 (1): 78-83.

24 R.R. Kulkarni, P.S. Patki, V.P. Jog, S.G. Gandage and Bhushan Patwardhan.
Treatment of osteoarthritis with a herbomineral formulation: a double-blind,
placebo-controlled, cross-over study. Journal of Ethnopharmacology (1991)
33: 91-95.

25 G.S.H. Ramakanth, C. Uday Kumar, P.V. Kishan, P. Usharni. A
randomized, double blind placebo controlled study of efficacy and tolerability
of Withania somnifera extracts in knee joint pain. Journal of Ayurveda and
Integrative Medicine (2016) 7: 151-157.

26 A. Mariappan, M. Devaprasad, Ashish Jaiswal, V. Banumathi, U.
Mabalirajan. Clinical evaluation of beneficial effects of Withania somnifera in
patients with rheumatoid arthritis: an open label single arm pilot study. World
Journal of Pharmacy and Pharmaceutical Sciences (2018) 7 (12): 743-767.

18 – Antimicrobial Activity

18.1 – Introduction

Since the introduction of penicillin in the early 1940s, antibiotics have been routinely used to treat infectious diseases. However, during the past few decades, many strains of antibiotic-resistant bacteria have evolved, posing a serious global health problem. According to a recent report from the World Health Organization, "Antibiotic-resistance is one of the biggest threats to global health, food security and development today"[1]. Actions to mitigate this problem have been suggested, including limiting the indiscriminate and inappropriate use of antibiotics. The potential of traditional medicinal plants as sources of antibacterial agents has received considerable attention. Extracts from various plants have been evaluated for antimicrobial activity. Results from studies evaluating the antimicrobial activity of Withania somnifera are summarized below.

18.2 – Summary of Results

Owais and coworkers[2] evaluated the antibacterial activity of various extracts of Withania somnifera (WS) against pathogenic bacteria. WS roots and leaves were separately extracted with hexane, ethyl acetate, methanol and water. All extracts except hexane showed antibacterial activity against E. coli, S. aureus and S. typhimurium. The methanol and water extracts were more effective than others. The methanol extract was subfractionated with ethyl acetate, n-butanol and water. All fractions showed activity against S. typhimurium, with the butanol fraction being most effective. Antibacterial activities of root and leaf extracts were also determined in Balb/c mice. Mice challenged with S. typhimurium died within 5 days. Mice challenged with S. typhimurium and treated with aqueous root or leaf extracts survived longer. Bacterial load in the liver and kidney on day 4 post-treatment was lower in extract-treated animals compared to untreated ones. The authors concluded that "The results from the present study are very encouraging and indicate this herb should be studied more extensively to explore its potential in the treatment of infectious diseases as well".

Mahesh and Satish[3] investigated the antimicrobial activity of a methanol extract of Withania somnifera roots and leaves against a number of bacteria (B. subtilis, E. coli, P. fluorescens, S. aureus and Xanthomonas axonopodis pv. malvacearum) and fungi (A. flavus, D. turcica and F. verticillioides). The extracts showed antimicrobial activity against all tested bacteria and fungi. The antibacterial activity was comparable to the standard streptomycin and antifungal activity to the standard nystatin.

Bhute and coworkers[4] reported the antibacterial activity of aqueous, alcoholic and chloroform extracts of Withania somnifera against two gram-positive (S. aureus and B. subtilis) and two gram-negative (P. aeruginosa and E. coli) bacteria. The effects of the aqueous extract and alcoholic extract did not differ much from each other, but the chloroform extract was found to be more effective in comparison.

Jain and Varshney[5] examined the antimicrobial activity of methanol and aqueous extracts of Withania somnifera roots against some gram-positive bacteria (Streptococcus mutans, Pseudomonas aeruginosa, Staphylococcus aureus), gram-negative bacteria (Escherichia coli) and a yeast (Candida albicans). Both extracts showed antimicrobial activity. The aqueous extract was more effective than the ethanol extract. The zone inhibition values for the bacteria ranged from 33 mm (S. aureus) to 50 mm (E. coli) for the aqueous extract and 15 mm (S. aureus) to 38 mm (E. coli, S. mutans) for the methanol extract. Zone inhibition values for the standard Ciprofloxacin ranged from 10 mm (P. Aeruginosa) to 35 mm (S. mutans). Zone inhibition values for C. albicans were 41 mm and 32 mm for the aqueous and methanol extracts respectively. The authors concluded that "the methanolic and aqueous root extracts of W. somnifera might be exploited as a natural drug for the treatment of several infectious diseases caused by these organisms".

Mehrotra and coworkers[6] reported the antibacterial activity of an aqueous extract of Withania somnifera roots against methicillin-resistant Staphylococcus aureus (MRSA). The antibacterial activity was retained over the temperature range 4-100 °C. TLC separation of the extract gave two spots. Spot 1 showed the presence of alkaloids and spot 2 showed the presence of essential oils and phenolics. The authors suggested that "the bioactive fractions separated from aqueous extract of W. somnifera is a potential source of antibacterial compounds with antioxidant property".

Singh and Kumar[7] evaluated the antibacterial activity of flavonoids from Withania somnifera against selected bacteria and fungi. Bound and free flavonoids were extracted separately from roots, stems, leaves and fruits of Withania somnifera and tested against the following pathogens:

- gram-positive bacteria: Staphylococcus aureus

- gram negative bacteria: Escherichia coli, Proteus mirabilis and Pseudomonas aeruginosa

- fungi: Candida albicans, Aspergillus flavus and Aspergillus niger

All extracts showed antimicrobial activity against one or more pathogens. C. albicans was the most susceptible, being subject to antibacterial activity by all extracts. Only bound flavonoids (flavonoids bound to a sugar moiety) extracted from roots showed antimicrobial activity against P. aeruginosa. The authors concluded that "Results of the present study reveal that extracts of W. somnifera showing great antimicrobial potential against test microorganisms may be exploited for future antimicrobial drugs".

Santhi and Swaminathan[8] evaluated the antibacterial activity of aqueous, alcoholic and acetone extracts of Withania somnifera leaves against S. aureus, E. coli, K. pneumoniae, P. aeruginosa, P. mirabilis and S. paratyphi. The acetone extract showed the highest antibacterial activity, followed by the ethanol extract. The aqueous extract showed less activity against most of the tested bacteria, but its antibacterial activity against P. mirabilis was greater than either acetone or alcohol. The authors concluded that "bioactive compounds from Withania somnifera leaf extracts could be used as an alternate to antibiotics, considering the side effects and escalating levels of antibiotic resistance among microorganisms".

Sundaram and coworkers[9] investigated the antibacterial activity of Withania somnifera extracts on some clinically isolated bacterial pathogens. Ethanol, ethyl acetate, dichloromethane and hexane extracts of Withania somnifera were tested against S. aureus, B. subtilis, E. coli and P. aeruginosa. All extracts exhibited antibacterial activity against all tested bacteria. Ethanol and ethyl acetate extracts showed strong activity, whereas dichloromethane and hexane extracts were not as effective.

Alam and coworkers[10] examined the antibacterial activity of methanol extracts of Withania somnifera leaves, fruits and roots against E. coli, S. typhi, C. freundii, P. aeruginosa and K. pneumoniae. All extracts exhibited antibacterial activity against all tested bacteria. Zone inhibition values for the root, fruit and leaf extracts ranged from 9.0 mm (P. aeruginosa) to 15 mm (E. coli), 8 mm (K.

pneumonia) to 14 mm (S. typhi) and 19.0 mm (K. pneumoniae) to 32 mm (S. typhi) respectively.

Singariya and coworkers[11] tested the antimicrobial activity of various extracts of Withania somnifera leaves against P. mirabilis, K. pneumoniae, A. tumefaciens and A. niger. Powdered leaves of Withania somnifera were sequentially extracted with hexane, petroleum ether, toluene, benzene, isopropyl alcohol, chloroform, ethyl acetate, acetone, ethanol, glacial acetic acid and water. All extracts exhibited antimicrobial activity against one or more microorganisms. The acetic acid extract was effective against all microorganisms tested and the chloroform extract was effective only against A. tumefaciens. In another similar investigation[12], extracts of Withania somnifera fruit coats (calyx) were tested against the same microorganisms. All extracts except benzene and hexane showed antimicrobial activity against one or more microorganisms. Singariya and coworkers[13] also examined the antimicrobial activity of different extracts of Withania somnifera roots, stems, leaves and flowers against P. aeruginosa, B. subtilis, E. aerogenes and A. flavus. The extracts were prepared by sequential extraction of Withania somnifera roots, stems, leaves and flowers separately with benzene, chloroform and water. Benzene extracts of roots, stems and leaves showed antimicrobial activity against P. aeruginosa and B. subtilis. Chloroform extracts of roots, stems and leaves showed activity against B. subtilis. Water extracts of roots, stems, leaves and flowers showed activity against P. aeruginosa. Singariya and coworkers[14] examined the antimicrobial activity of various extracts of ripened fruits of Withania somnifera. Ripened fruits of Withania somnifera were powdered and extracted sequentially with hexane, petroleum ether, toluene, benzene, isopropyl alcohol, chloroform, ethyl acetate, acetone, glacial acetic acid and water. The extracts were tested against P. mirabilis, K. pneumoniae, A. tumefaciens and A. niger. All extracts showed antimicrobial activity against one or more microorganisms, indicating broad spectrum antimicrobial activity of Withania somnifera.

Rizwana and coworkers[15] evaluated the antibacterial activity of acetone, ethanol, methanol and chloroform extracts of Withania somnifera leaves, stems and roots against a number of human pathogenic bacteria: B. subtilis, methicillin-resistant S. aureus (MRSA), S. pyogenes, E. faecalis, E. coli, P. aeruginosa and K. pneumoniae. Acetone extracts of leaves, stems and roots were effective against all bacteria tested. Other extracts were effective against most of the bacteria tested. Extracts and bacteria against which they showed no effect are listed below:

- Methanol extracts of stems and leaves: no effect on MRSA and K. pneumoniae

- Ethanol extract of leaves: no effect on K. pneumoniae
- Chloroform extract of stems: no effect on P. aeruginosa
- Chloroform extract of roots: no effect on MRSA, S. pyogenes, E. coli and P. aeruginosa

The authors concluded that "acetone, methanolic and ethanolic extracts of W. somnifera might be exploited as natural drug for the treatment of several infectious diseases caused by these organisms".

Adaikkappan and coworkers[16] demonstrated the anti-mycobacterial activity of an aqueous extract of Withania somnifera leaves and roots against Mycobacterium tuberculosis $H_{37}Rv$. (M.TB). Treatment of M.TB with the extract (0.01–1.0 mg/mL) showed dose-dependent inhibition of M.TB growth.

Pujari and coworkers[17] examined the antibacterial activity of water, ethanol and chloroform extracts of Withania somnifera roots against S. aureus, S. typhi and S. dysenteriae. Extracts were of two forms, crude and membrane-filtered. None of the extracts showed antibacterial activity against S. dysenteriae. Crude ethanol and chloroform extracts showed activity against S. aureus and S. typhi. The membrane-filtered chloroform extract showed activity only against S. aureus. The membrane-filtered water extract showed no activity against any of the bacteria tested.

Singh and Kumar[18] tested the antibacterial activity of alkaloid extracts of Withania somnifera roots, stems, fruits and leaves against E. aerogenes, B. subtilis, K. pneumoniae, R. planticola and A. tumefaciens. The root extract showed activity against all five bacteria, with Inhibition zone (IZ) values ranging from 8.75 mm (B. subtilis) to 15.25 mm (A, tumefaciens). The stem extract showed activity against all bacteria except R. planticola, with IZ values ranging from 8.25 mm (B. subtilis) to 25.5 mm (E. aerogenes). The leaf extract showed activity against all bacteria except B. subtilis, with IZ values ranging from 8.75 mm (R. planticola) to 15.75 mm (K. pneumoniae). The fruit extract showed activity only against R. planticola (IZ = 9.75 mm) and A. tumefaciens (IZ = 11.75 mm). The authors concluded that "studied plant is potentially a good source of antibacterial agents".

Sinha[19] examined the antibacterial activity of methanol, ethanol and water extracts of Withania somnifera roots, stems and leaves against S. aureus, B. subtilis, M. luteus, E. coli, P. aeruginosa, S. dysenteriae, S. flexneri and V. cholerae. Aqueous extracts of roots, stems and leaves showed no activity against any of the tested bacteria. The methanol root extract showed activity against all tested bacteria, with IZ values ranging from 8 mm (V. cholerae) to 16 mm (M. luteus).

The methanol leaf extract showed activity against all tested bacteria, with IZ values ranging from 8 mm (V. cholerae, S. flexneri) to 17 mm (M. luteus). The methanol stem extract showed activity against all bacteria except S. flexneri and V. cholerae, with IZ values ranging from 8 mm (S. dysenteriae) to 12 mm (B. subtilis, M. luteus). The ethanol leaf extract showed activity against all tested bacteria, with IZ values ranging from 8 mm (S. dysenteriae, S. flexneri, V. cholerae) to 16 mm (M. luteus). The ethanol root extract showed activity against all tested bacteria, with IZ values ranging from 8 mm (S. flexneri, V. cholerae) to 15 mm (M. luteus). The ethanol stem extract showed activity against all tested bacteria except S. flexneri and V. cholerae, with IZ values ranging from 8 mm (P. aeruginosa, S. dysenteriae) to 10 mm (B. subtilis, M. luteus).

Halmova and coworkers[20] tested the antibacterial activity of an acetone extract of Withania somnifera aerial parts against some human pathogenic bacteria (B. cereus, B. subtilis, S. aureus, S. epidermis, S. pneumoniae and S. pyogenes) and bifidobacteria (B. animalis, B. breve, B. catenulatum, B. infantis and B. longum). The extract showed activity against all tested bacteria, but it was more effective against human pathogenic bacteria. IZ values for human pathogenic bacteria ranged from 14.3 mm (B. cereus) to 25.0 mm (S. epidermis), with an average value of 20.45 mm. The average value for the standard vancomycin was 17.45 mm. IZ values for bifidobacteria ranged from 9.45 mm (B. animalis) to 17.0 mm (B. infantis), with an average value of 13.1 mm. The average value of the standard vancomycin was 21.2 mm. The authors concluded that "These results suggest W. somnifera as an effective antibacterial agent against human pathogenic bacteria with lowered harmful effect on bifidobacteria".

Jamal and coworkers[21] examined the antibacterial activity of water and ethanol extracts of Withania somnifera leaves and fruits against B. subtilis, E. coli, S. aureus and S. epidermitis. The ethanol leaf extract showed no activity against any of the tested bacteria. The water leaf extract showed activity against all tested bacteria, with IZ values ranging from 15.2 mm (B. subtilis) to 20.2 mm (E. coli). Both the ethanol and water fruit extracts showed activity against all tested bacteria. IZ values for the ethanol extract ranged from 16.2 mm (S. aureus) to 17.1 mm (E. coli) and for the water extract from 21.2 mm (S. aureus) to 28.1 mm (B. subtilis). IZ values for the standard gentamicin ranged from 24 mm (S. aureus, E. coli) to 26.0 mm (S. epidermitis).

Jeyanthi and coworkers[22] made a comparative study of the antibacterial activity of ethanol and methanol extracts of Withania somnifera roots with standard antibiotics. The extracts were tested against B.

subtilis, E. coli, K. pneumoniae, P. aeruginosa and S. paratyphi. Both extracts showed activity against all tested bacteria, with the methanol extract being more effective. IZ values for the methanol extract ranged from 16 mm (B. subtilis) to 22 mm (P. aeruginosa) and for the ethanol extract from 14 mm (B. subtilis) to 19 mm (P. aeruginosa). IZ values for the standard tetracycline ranged from 14 mm (B. subtilis) to 20 mm (P. aeruginosa) and for gentamicin from 11 mm (B. subtilis) to 21 mm (P. aeruginosa, S. paratyphi). The authors concluded that the "methanol root extract of W. somnifera with its well-powered bioactive compounds can counteract these bacterial strains, which direct the human life towards the valuable traditional medicine against the drug resistant microbes".

Al-Ani and coworkers[23] investigated the antibacterial activity of aqueous, ethanol and acetone extracts of Withania somnifera leaves against S. aureus, E. coli, K. pneumoniae, P. aeruginosa, P. mirabilis and S. paratyphi B. All extracts showed activity against all tested bacteria. IZ values for the aqueous extract ranged from 5 mm (S. paratyphi B) to 27 mm (K. pneumoniae); for the ethanol extract, from 2 mm (P. aeruginosa) to 25 mm (K. pneumoniae); and for the acetone extract, from 4 mm (P. aeruginosa) to 16 mm (S. aureus). IZ values for the standard gentamicin ranged from 18 mm (S. aureus, E. coli) to 28 mm (K. pneumoniae). The authors concluded that "our findings suggest that an appropriate bioactive compound may be developed from leaves of Withania somnifera (L.) as an alternate to antibiotics".

Mwitari and coworkers[24] sequentially extracted aerial parts of Withania somnifera with hexane, dichloromethane, ethyl acetate and methanol, and tested their antimicrobial activity. The dichloromethane and ethyl acetate extracts showed activity against S. aureus and MRSA. They also showed showed some activity against Microsporum gypseum and Trichophyton mentagrophytes.

Mali and Singh[25] isolated Withanolide A from Withania somnifera stems and demonstrated its antibacterial activity against Pseudomonas and Staphylococcus aureus.

Bashir and coworkers[26] examined the antibacterial activity of a methanol extract of Withania somnifera and three flavonoids isolated from the extract. The extract and the flavonoids showed moderate activity against B. subtilis, E. coli, N. gonorrhoeae, P. aeruginosa and S. aureus.

Ramachandran and Kumar[27] examined the antimicrobial activity of an ethanol extract of Withania somnifera stems against E. coli, S. typhi, K. pneumoniae, A. niger and T. viride. The extract showed activity against all microorganisms. Zone inhibition values ranged between 16 mm (S. typhi) to 18 mm (E. coli, A. niger).

Bisht and Rawat[28] reported the antibacterial activity of a methanol extract of Withania somnifera leaves against MRSA, MSSA, Enterococcus and Streptococcus spp. IZ values were close to 20 mm.

Singh and Kumar[29] tested the antimicrobial activity of flavonoid extracts of Withania somnifera leaves, stems, roots and fruits against E. aerogenes, B. subtilis, K. pneumoniae, R. Planticola and A. tumefaciens. All extracts showed antimicrobial activity against at least two of the microorganisms. Bound flavonoids were found to be more effective than free flavonoids. Bound flavonoids of stems and roots showed activity against all five microorganisms.

Dharajiya and coworkers[30] tested the antimicrobial activity of hexane, ethyl acetate, methanol and water extracts of Withania somnifera against gram-positive bacteria (B. cereus), gram-negative bacteria (E. coli, S. marcescens and P. aeruginosa) and fungi (A. niger, A. flavus, A. oryzae, P. chrysogenum and T. viride). The methanol and water extracts showed activity against all tested bacteria. IZ for the methanol extract ranged from 9.5 mm (P. aeruginosa) to 17.67 mm (E. coli) and for the aqueous extract from 8.33 mm (B. cereus) to 11.33 mm (E coli). The hexane extract showed activity against S. marcescens (IZ = 12.0 mm) and B. cereus (IZ = 8.5mm). The ethyl acetate extract showed activity against S. marcescens (IZ = 8.33 mm). The hexane, ethyl acetate, methanol and aqueous extracts showed antifungal activity against T. viride with IZ values of 8.67 mm, 9.83 mm, 10.0 mm and 8.50 mm respectively.

Soni and coworkers[31] examined the antibacterial activity of methanol and ethanol extracts of Withania somnifera leaves against S. aureus, B. subtilis, P. vulgaris and P. aeruginosa. Both extracts showed activity against all tested bacteria. The methanol extract showed IZ values of 21 mm, 20 mm, 22 mm, and 20 mm for S. aureus, B. subtilis, P. vulgaris and P. aeruginosa respectively. The ethanol extract showed IZ values of 20 mm, 24 mm, 22 mm and 20 mm for S. aureus, B. subtilis, P. vulgaris and P. aeruginosa respectively.

Bahadar and coworkers[32] examined the antibacterial activity of an ethanol extract of Withania somnifera against E. coli, P. aeruginosa, Salmonella spp, Klebsiella spp and S. aureus. IZ values ranged from 10 mm (Klebsiella spp) to 20 mm (E. coli). The standard ampicillin showed IZ values ranging from 10 mm (Klebsiella spp) to 38 mm (E. coli).

Kharel and coworkers[33] isolated a withanolide (WS-1) from a methanol extract of Withania somnifera and tested its antibacterial activity against B. subtilis, K. pneumoniae, S aureus, E. coli, P. vulgaris, P. aeruginosa and S. typhi. WS-1 showed antibacterial activity against all tested bacteria. IZ values ranged from 8.33 mm (P. vulgaris) to 20.66 mm (K. pneumoniae).

Zaynab and Fatemeh[34] reported the antibacterial activity of an aqueous extract of Withania somnifera leaves against S. aureus, S. pyogenes, S. pneumoniae, H. alvei, S. saprophyticus, A. baumannii, E. faecalis, P. mirabilis and S. marcescens. The extract was more effective against S. pneumoniae than the others.

Bokaeian and coworkers[35] showed the antibacterial activity of an ethanol extract of Withania somnifera leaves against antibiotic- (ceftazidime, cefixime, erythromycin) resistant isolates of K. pneumoniae. In another study, Bokaeian and Saeidi[36] demonstrated the antibacterial activity of an ethanol extract of Withania somnifera leaves against antibiotic- (oxacillin, ceftazidime, penicillin, trimethoprim-sulfamethoxazole, cefixime, vancomycin) resistant isolates of S. aureus.

Muddukrishnaiah and Singh[37] showed the antimicrobial activity of aqueous and alcohol extracts of Withania somnifera rhizomes against a number of multidrug-resistant strains of S. aureus, P. aeruginosa, K. pneumoniae, P. vulgaris and E. coli. IZ values for the ethanol extract ranged from 12 mm to 23 mm and for the aqueous extract from 12 mm to 17 mm.

References

1   Antibiotic Resistance, World Health Organization. https://www.who.int/news-room/fact-sheets/detail/antibiotic-resistance
2   M. Owais, K. S. Sharad, A. Shehbaz, M. Saleemuddin. Antibacterial efficacy of Withania somnifera (ashwagandha) an indigenous medicinal plant against experimental murine salmonellosis. Phytomedicine (2005) 12: 229-235.
3   B. Mahesh and S. Satish. Antimicrobial activity of some important medicinal plants against plant and human pathogens. World Journal of Agricultural Sciences (2008) 4(S): 839-843.
4   Bhute Shrikant S, Kukreja Girish P, Godse Varsha V, Kshirsagar Jayant K. In vitro antibacterial activity of Withania somnifera (Ashwagandha) root extract. Adv Pharmacol Toxicol (2010) 11 (1): 65-69.
5   Pranay Jain and Rishabh Varshney. Antimicrobial activity of aqueous and methanolic extracts of Withania somnifera (Ashwagandha). Journal of Chemical and Pharmaceutical Research (2011) 3 (3): 260-263.
6   Vidhi Mehrotra, Shubhi Mehrotra, Vandna Kirar, Radhey Shyam, Kshipra Misra, Ashwani Kumar Srivastava, Shoma Paul Nandi. Antioxidant and anti microbial activities of aqueous extract of Withania somnifera against methicillin-resistant Staphylococcus aureus. Journal of Microbiology and Biotechnology Research (2011) 1(1): 40-45.
7   G. Singh and P. Kumar. Evaluation of antimicrobial efficacy of flavonoids of Withania somnifera L. Indian Journal of Pharmaceutical Sciences (2011) 73

(4): 473-478.
8   Santhi M and Swaminathan C. Evaluation of antibacterial activity and phytochemical analysis of leaves of Withania somnifera (L.) Dunal, International Journal of Current Research (2011) 3 (3): 10-12.
9   Shanthy Sundaram, Priyanka Dwivedi and Shalini Purwar. In vitro evaluation of antibacterial activities of crude extracts of Withania somnifera (Ashwagandha) to bacterial pathogens. Asian Journal of Biotechnology (2011) 3 (2): 194-199.
10   Nadia Alam, Monzur Hossain, Md Abdul Mottalib, Siti Amrah Sulaiman, Siew Hua Gan and Md Ibrahim Khalil. Methanolic extracts of Withania somnifera leaves, fruits and roots possess antioxidant properties and antibacterial activities. BMC Complementary and Alternative Medicine (2012) 12: 175.
11   Premlata Singariya, Padma Kumar and Krishan Kumar Mourya. Evaluation of antimicrobial activity of leaf extracts of winter cherry (Withania somnifera). International Journal of Pharm Tech Research (2012) 4 (3): 1247-1253.
12   Premlata Singariya, Padma Kumar and Krishan Kumar Mourya. Antimicrobial activity of fruit coat (calyx) of Withania somnifera against some multidrug resistant microbes. International Journal of Biological & Pharmaceutical Research (2012) 3 (2): 252-258.
13   P Singariya, P Kumar and K K Mourya. Comparative primary phyto-profile and microbial activity of Cenchrus ciliaris (Anjan grass) and Withania somnifera (Winter cherry). IJRAP (2012) 3(2): 303-308.
14   Premalata Singariya, Padma Kumar and Krishan Kumar Mourya. Ripen fruits of Indian ginseng: Phyto-chemical and pharmacological examination against human and plant pathogens. International Journal of Applied Biology and Pharmaceutical Technology (2012) 3 (2): 1-8.
15   Humaira Rizwana, Amal Abdulaziz Al Hazzani, Afaf Ibrahim Shehata and Nadine Mohamed Safouh Moubayed. Antibacterial potential of Withania somnifera L. against human pathogenic bacteria. African Journal of Microbiology Research (2012) 6 (22): 4810-4815.
16   Periyakaruppan Adaikkappan, Manickavasagam Kannapiran and Arulandhu Anthonisamy. Anti-mycobacterial activity of Withania somnifera and Pueraria tuberosa against Mycobacterium tuberculosis H$_{37}$Rv. J. Acad, Indus. Res (2012) 1(4):153-156.
17   Pujari S. A. and Gandhi M. B. Studies on effect of root extracts of Withania somnifera on some clinically isolated bacterial pathogens. Journal of Environmental Research and Development (2012) 7 (2A): 1032-1035.
18   Geeta Singh and Padma Kumar. Antibacterial potential of alkaloids of Withania somnifera L. & Euphorbia hirta L. International Journal of Pharmacy and Pharmaceutical Sciences (2012) 4 (1): 78-81.
19   Sankar Narayan Sinha. Screening of antioxidant and antibacterial activities of various extracts of Withania somnifera (L.) Dunal. International Journal of Pharmacology and Therapeutics (2012) 2 (1): 36-42.
20   K. Halamova, L. Kokoska, Z. Polesny, K. Macakova, J. Flesar and V. Rada. Selective in vitro growth inhibitory effect of Withania somnifera on human pathogenic bacteria and bifidobacteria. Pak. J. Bot (2013) 45 (2): 667-670.
21   Qaiser Jamal, Shahzad Munir, Sikandar Khan Sherwani, Mohammad Sualeh, Uzma Jabeen, Muhammad Saqib Malik, Mubashir Hussain. Antibacterial activity of two medicinal plants: Withania somnifera and Curcumin longa. European Academic Research (2013) 1(6): 1335-1345.
22   T. Jeyanthi, P. Subramanian, P. Kumaravel. A comparative analysis of antibacterial activity of Withania somnifera root extract with commercial antibiotics. Asian J. Pharm. Res (2013) 3 (2): 98-102.

23 Nabeel Al-Ani, Sabreen A. Hadi, Rawaa Nazar. Antimicrobial activities of Withania somnifera crude extract. Scientia Agriculture (2013) 4 (3): 74-76.

24 Peter G. Mwitari, Peter A. Ayeka, Joyce Ondicho, Esther N. Matu, Christine C. Bii. Antimicrobial activity and probable mechanisms of action of medicinal plants of Kenya: Withania somnifera, Warbugia ugandensis, Prunus africana and Plectrunthus barbatus. PLOSS ONE June 2013, vol3. Issue 6. e65619.

25 Pratap Chand Mali and Ashish Ranjan Singh. Isolation, characterization and evaluation of antimicrobial activity of Withanolide-A of Withania somnifera. International Journal of Pharmacological Research (2013) 3 (3): 48-52.

26 Bashir H. S., Mohammed A. M, Magsoud A.S., Shaoub A. M. Isolation of three flavonoids from Withania somnifera leaves (Solanaceae) and their antimicrobial activities. Journal of Forest Products and Industries (2013) 2 (5): 39-45.

27 A. Ramachandran and M. Senthil Kumar. FT-IR, UV and antimicrobial activity Withania somnifera and Withania Obtusifolia. International Journal of Pharma and Bio Sciences (2014) 5 (4): 111-117.

28 Punum Bisht, Vinita Rawat. Antibacterial activity of Withania somnifera against gram-positive isolates from pus samples. AYU (2014) 35 (3): 330-332.

29 Geeta Singh, Padma Kumar. Antibacterial activity of flavonoids of Withania somnifera L. International Journal of Green Pharmacy (2014) 8 (2): 114-118.

30 Darshan Dharajiya, Payal Patel, Mamta Patel, Nupur Moitra. In vitro antimicrobial activity and qualitative phytochemical analysis of Withania somnifera (L.) Dunal extracts. Int. J. Pharm. Sci. Rev. Res (2014) 27 (2): 349-354.

31 Prerna Soni, A. N. Bahadur, U. Tewari. Study on antimicrobial activity of leaf extract of Withania somnifera L. Dunal against clinical pathogens. Int. J. Adv. Res. Biol. Sci (2015) 2 (11): 193-196.

32 Sulaiman Bahadar, Khalil U Rahman, Muhammad Daud, Fahad Ali, ILyas Khan, Hizbullah Noreen Akhtar, Rabia Zardad, Usman Kamal, Komal Habib, Irfan Ullah, Abdul Majeed, Azam Hayat and Mujaddad-ur-Rehman. Medicinal activity of Withania somnifera and Otostegia limbata against selected pathogens. American-Eurasian J. Agric. & Environ. Sci (2015) 15 (9): 1849-1853.

33 Prakash Kharel, Mangala D. Manandhar, Surya K. Kalauni. Suresh Awale and Janaki Baral. Isolation, identification and antimicrobial activity of a Withanolide [WS-1] from the roots of Withania somnifera. Nepal Journal of Science and Technology (2011) 12: 179-186.

34 Mohkami Zaynab and Bidarnamani Fatemeh. Evaluation of antimicrobial activity of Withania somnifera aqueous extract against human pathogens. Indian Journal of Fundamental and Applied Life Sciences (2014) 4 (S4): 2969-2973.

35 Mohammad Bokaeian, Saeidi Saeidi, Zahra Shahi, Shahla Sahraei, Hemadollah Zarei, Gelareh Sohil Baigi. Evaluation of antibacterial activity of Withania somnifera leaf extracts against antibiotic-resistant isolates of Klebsiella pneumoniae. Int J Infect (2014) 1(2): e21085.

36 Mohammad Bokaeian, Saeide Saeidi. Evaluation of antimicrobial activity of leaf extract of Withania somnifera against antibiotic resistant Staphylococcus aureus. Zahedan J Res Med Sci (2015) 17 (7):e1016.

37 Muddukrishnaiah K and Sumita Singh. Antimicrobial, synergistic activity and antioxidant studies on multidrug resistance human pathogen using crude extract of Azadirachta indica leaf and Withania somnifera rhizome. J Plant Pathol Microbiol (2015). S3: 009. doi: 10.4172/2157-7471.S3-009

19 – Reproductive System Protective Activities

19.1 – Introduction

Infertility is a global concern. A study found that in 2010, about 50 million couples were unable to have a child after trying for years. The study also pointed out that infertility rates remained relatively unchanged for 20 years (1990-2010)[1]. Infertility is a complex, heterogeneous disorder that can result from issues with the male partner, female partner or both. Various safe and effective techniques are available for the treatment of infertility. Withania somnifera is one of the major medicinal plants used in ayurveda[2,3] to treat sexual disorders and infertility. A number of animal studies and a few with human subjects have shown its effectiveness, and the results from some studies are summarized below.

Al-Qarawi and coworkers[4] showed that treating immature female Wistar rats with an aqueous extract of Withania somnifera (47 mg/100 g/day, via stomach tube) for 6 days increased ovarian weight and caused significant changes in LH and FSH compared to controls. Histological examination of ovaries showed growing follicles with well-developed granulosa.

Abdel-Magied and coworkers[5] evaluated the effect of an aqueous extract of Withania somnifera leaves (WS) on testicular development in immature male Wistar rats. The following observations were made in rats treated with WS (47 mg/100 g/day, via stomach tube) for six days compared to controls:

- increased testicular weight
- increased diameter of seminiferous tubules as well as increased seminiferous tubular cell layers in the testis
- decreased serum testosterone and FSH and increased ICSH

The authors concluded that "W. somnifera induces testicular development and spermatogenesis in immature Wistar rats by directly affecting the seminiferous tubules".

Kiasalari and coworkers[6] examined the effect of Withania somnifera root powder (WS) on sex hormones in diabetic rats. Adult male Wistar rats were injected with streptozotocin to induce diabetes. Diabetic rats given a diet containing WS for four weeks showed increased serum progesterone, testosterone and LH, decreased serum FSH, and no change in serum estrogen compared to diabetic rats given a normal diet. The authors concluded that "Our study has indicated that long time oral administration of somnifera root in experimental model of streptozotocin-induced diabetes, could be used as a good candidate in the treatment of reproductive hormones deficiency".

Rajashree and coworkers[7] examined the effect of an alcoholic (70%) extract of Withania somnifera roots (WS) on reproductive organs in diabetic rats. Diabetes was induced in adult male albino rats (60 days old) by injecting a single dose of streptozotocin (50 mg/kg, i.p.). At the end of the experimental period (30 days), diabetic rats showed a decreased body weight, Cauda epididymis weight and sperm count compared to controls. Treatment of diabetic rats with insulin (5 units/kg/day, i.p.) or WS (500 mg/ kg/day. P.O.) for 30 days showed a reversal of these changes. WS was more effective than insulin. The authors concluded that "Withania somnifera root extracts had the potency to increase the reproductive efficacy of the diabetic rats".

Kyathanahalli and coworkers[8] investigated the effect of a Withania somnifera root extract (WS) on diabetes-induced testicular oxidative impairments in prepubertal rats. Diabetes was induced in prepubertal male CFT-Wistar rats by injecting a single dose of streptozotocin (90 mg/kg, i.p.). At the end of the experimental period, the following observations were made in diabetic rats compared to controls:

- increased LPO, ROS, GST and GR, and decreased CAT, GPx and total thiol content in testis mitochondria and cytosol
- increased GSH and SOD in testis mitochondria

Diabetic rats treated with WS (500 mg/kg/day, via oral gavage) for 15 days reversed these changes. Diabetic rats also showed increased LDH and G6PDH, and decreased levels of 3β-HSD in the testis compared to controls. Diabetic rats treated with WS showed a reversal of these changes. The authors concluded that "oral supplementation of WS may be considered as an auxiliary therapy together with conventional medicines to improve the secondary complications associated with diabetes".

Belal and coworkers[9] investigated the effect of Withania somnifera root powder (WS) on the levels of sex hormones in diabetic and non-diabetic rats. Diabetes was induced in adult male albino Wistar rats by injecting a single dose of alloxan (150 mg/kg, S.C.). Normal rats treated with a diet containing WS (6.25%) for four weeks showed increased serum progesterone, testosterone and LH, decreased serum FSH and no change in serum estrogen compared to normal rats treated with the regular diet. Similar observations were made in diabetic rats treated with a diet containing WS compared to diabetic rats treated with a regular diet.

Kumar and coworkers[10] examined the effect of an aqueous extract of Withania somnifera roots (WS) on LPO, sperm count and seminiferous tubules in mice exposed to endosulfan (an organochlorine insecticide). Swiss albino mice were treated with endosulfan for four weeks or treated with endosulfan for four weeks followed by WS for four weeks. Mice treated with distilled water served as controls. Mice treated with endosulfan showed increased serum LPO and a decreased semen sperm count compared to controls. Mice treated with endosulfan followed by WS showed an increased sperm count and decreased LPO compared to the endosulfan group. Seminiferous tubules of the endosulfan group showed degenerated interstitial space and clustered primary and secondary spermatocytes. The endosulfan+WS group showed restoration in seminiferous tubules. The authors concluded that "Withania somnifera causes restoration in biochemical and histological parameters and restores normal sperm count in male mice".

Kumar and coworkers[11] also found that treating Swiss female albino mice with the organophosphate insecticide chlorpyrifos (6 mg/kg/day, via gavage) for 8 weeks increased serum estrogen and cholesterol and caused ovary alterations compared to controls. Treatment of mice with chlorpyrifos for 8 weeks followed by treatment with an alcohol extract of Withania somnifera roots (50 mg/kg/day) or a rhizome extract of Curcuma longa (50 mg/kg/day) for 8 weeks reversed the changes in cholesterol and estrogen as well as mitigated the ovary changes induced by chlorpyrifos. Withania somnifera was more effective than Curcuma longa. The authors concluded that "Withania somnifera and Curcuma longa both play effective role against Chlorpyrifos induced toxicity on biochemical, hormonal and histology of ovary, however Withania somnifera has great restorative effect against Chlorpyrifos induced toxicity than Curcuma longa comparatively".

Jasuja and coworkers[12] investigated the effects of an ethanol (70%) extract of Withania somnifera leaves and roots (WS) on acephate (an organophosphate insecticide)-induced sex hormonal changes in rats. Fertile male albino rats treated with acephate (7.5 mg/kg/day) for 30 days showed decreased serum testosterone, LH and FSH compared to controls. Rats treated with acephate (7.5 mg/kg/day) and WS (100 mg/kg/day) for 30 days showed a reduction of the changes induced by acephate. Testes in the control group showed a normal seminiferous tubule histoarchitecture with all the successive stages of spermatogenesis. Testes in the acephate group showed irregular seminiferous tubules with inhibited spermatogenesis. Testes in the acephate+WS group showed attenuation of the changes induced by acephate. The authors concluded that "oral administration of W. somnifera extract could prevent or be helpful in reducing the complications of reproductive toxicity associated with oxidative stress".

Patil and coworkers[13] examined the spermatogenic activity of an ethanol extract of Withania somnifera leaves (WS) in mice subjected to D-galactose-induced oxidative stress. Male albino mice were treated for 15 days with sterile water, 5% D-galactose or 5% D-galactose+2% WS. The mice were sacrificed and the testis and epididymis were excised for analysis. The D-galactose group showed increased total LPO, increased mitochondrial peroxidation and a decreased sperm count compared to controls. The D-galactose+WS group showed decreased total LPO, decreased mitochondrial peroxidation and an increased sperm count compared to the D-galactose group. Histological examination of testes in the D-galactose group showed a highly disorganized structure of seminiferous tubules and fewer sperms in the lumen compared to controls. Histological examination of the epididymis in the D-galactose group showed alterations compared to controls. The D-galactose+WS group showed no significant histological changes compared to controls. The authors concluded that "The overall findings may be helpful to the population not only to treat infertility but also to maintain normal sex life".

Shaikh and coworkers[14] examined the effect of glycowithanolides (WSG) on D-galactose-induced oxidative damage to the testes and accessory reproductive organs in mice. Swiss albino male mice injected with a 5% solution of D-galactose (0.5 ml/day, S.C.) for 20 days showed decreased SOD, CAT, and GPx in the testes, epididymis and seminal vesicles compared to controls. Mice treated with D-galactose (0.5 ml/day, S.C.) along with WSG (20 mg/kg/day) for 20 days and mice treated with D-galactose (0.5 ml/day, S.C.) for 20 days followed by treatment with WSG (20 mg/kg/day) for 20 days showed a reversal of these changes. Histological studies[15] of the testes of mice treated with D-galactose showed fewer spermatogonia, spermatocytes, spermatids and Leydig cells compared to controls, indicating the anti-spermatogenic effects of D-galactose. Treatment with WSG mitigated the effects of D-galactose. Histological studies also showed that D-galactose caused major morphological changes in the epididymis and seminal vesicles, and treatment with WSG mitigated the effects.

Kaspate and coworkers[16] reported that a hydroalcoholic extract of Withania somnifera roots (WS) increased sexual activity in female Wistar rats. Tubal ligated rats treated with WS (100-300 mg/kg/day, P.O.) for 21 days showed increased sexual behaviors as measured by the automated runway and copulatory arena apparatuses compared to controls. The genital organ histology of WS-treated animals was normal.

Rahamati and coworkers[17] examined the effect of Withania somnifera root powder (WS) on sex hormones and gonadotropin levels in morphine-addicted male rats. Male rats treated with morphine for 21 days showed significantly decreased plasma levels of estrogen, testosterone and LH, a slightly decreased level of progesterone, and a slightly increased level of FSH compared to controls. Rats treated with morphine+WS (incorporated in the diet) for 21 days showed significantly increased levels of estrogen, testosterone and LH, a slightly increased level of progesterone, and no significant change in FSH compared to morphine-treated rats.

Kumar and coworkers[18] studied the effect of an alcohol (70%) extract of Withania somnifera roots (WS) on arsenic-induced testicular toxicity in rats. Charles Foster rats treated with sodium arsenite (8 mg/kg/day, P.O.) for 45 days showed the following changes compared to controls:

- nausea, nose bleeding, lack of body coordination and weakness
- decreased sperm count and sperm motility
- decreased serum testosterone, increased LH and increased LPO
- degeneration of sperm morphology and complete arrest of spermatogenetic stages

Rats treated with sodium arsenite for 45 days followed by treatment with WS (100 mg/kg/day) for 30 days showed a reversal of these changes. The authors concluded that "W. somnifera is the novel drug which not only possesses antioxidant and rejuvenating property but also maintains the cellular integrity of testicular cells leading to normal functioning".

Prithviraj and coworkers[19] examined the effect of Withania somnifera root powder (WS) on cadmium-induced oxidative injury in rat testes. Male Wistar albino rats were treated with a single dose of Cd (2.5 mg/kg, i.p.), a single dose of Cd (2.5 mg/kg, i.p.) followed by WS (1000 mg/kg/day, via gavage) for 30 days, or a single dose of Cd (2.5 mg/kg, i.p.) followed by vitamin E (300 mg/kg/day, via gavage) for 30 days. Untreated rats were used as controls. The following observations were made on testes in the Cd group compared to controls:

- decreased weight and volume
- increased ROS and LPO, and decreased enzymatic and non-enzymatic antioxidants
- necrotic changes in the seminiferous epithelium and increased apoptotic cells per tubule
- decreased activated caspase-3
- upregulation of iNOS expression and downregulation of MnSOD

Treatment of Cd-injected rats with WS or vitamin E mitigated these changes. The authors stated that "W. somnifera root may prove to be useful in treating/preventing oxidative stress and/or inflammatory related ailments and merit further research on male related infertility with redox and inflammation".

Saritha and coworkers[20] showed that Withania somnifera (WS) can mitigate reproductive alterations in female rats caused by lead exposure during the perinatal period. Rats were given lead acetate in drinking water from gestation day 1 through pregnancy, delivery and completion of the lactation period. Female pups were separated and fed a normal diet or a WS-incorporated diet for 45 days. After estrus cycles were checked, they were cohabited with normal male rats. Rats fed with the normal diet showed a longer diestrus phase, fewer implantations, fewer corpora lutea and fewer live fetuses compared to controls. The WS-treated group showed mitigation of these changes. The authors concluded that "exposure to Pb during perinatal period suppresses the female fertility and the reformulated diet with supplementation of Withania somnifera ameliorates Pb-induced female reproductive toxicity".

Bhargavan and coworkers[21] found that an alcohol (95%) extract of Withania somnifera roots (WSEE) prevented alcohol-induced testicular toxicity in rats. Adult male albino rats were treated with distilled water (control group), alcohol (4 g/kg/day, P.O.), or WSEE (200 mg/kg/day, P.O.) followed by alcohol (4 g/kg/day, P.O.) after 4 hours for 28 days. The following observations were made in the alcohol only group compared to the control group:

- decreased body and testes weight
- decreased sperm count and motility and increased sperm abnormality
- increased MDA and decreased CAT and GSH
- significant histological changes in the testes

The WSEE+alcohol group showed a reversal of these changes. The authors concluded that "WS appears as a promising candidate in preventing the alcohol induced testicular toxicity".

Divyashree and Yajurvedi[22] examined the effect of an alcohol extract of Withania somnifera roots (WS) on stress-induced alterations in rat ovaries. Adult female Wistar rats subjected to restraint stress (1 h/day) followed by forced swimming (15 min/day) for 28 days showed the following changes compared to controls (rats treated with the vehicle and not subjected to stress):

- decreased percentage gain in body weight
- increased relative adrenal gland weight and 3β-HSDH activity
- decreased relative ovarian weight and 3β-HSDH activity
- increased serum corticosterone concentration
- increased MDA concentration and decreased activities of SOD, CAT, GST and GPx in ovarian homogenate
- decreased mean healthy antral follicles and percentage of healthy granulosa cells
- increased atretic antral follicles and apoptotic ovarian granulosa cells

Rats treated with WS (10 mg/kg/day, P.O.) followed by the same stress regimen for 28 days showed a reversal of these changes. The authors concluded that "The present study shows the efficacy of alcoholic extract of Ashwagandha root in maintaining the normal ovarian functions despite stress experienced by the rats".

Ilayperuma and coworkers[23] examined the effect of a methanol extract of Withania somnifera roots (WS) on the sexual competence of male rats. Adult male Wistar rats were placed in separate cages and treated with WS (3000 mg/kg/day, P.O.) for 7 days. An estrous female rat was placed in each cage on certain days during and after treatment. The WS-treated group showed impaired libido, reduced

sexual vigor and performance and penile erectile dysfunction compared to controls. The effects were partially reversed after termination of the treatment. The authors concluded that "use of W.
somnifera may be detrimental to male sexual performance".

Singh and coworkers[24] found that an ethanol extract of Withania
somnifera stems was spermicidal and produced infertility in male
albino rats.

Mali[25] observed that a hydroalcoholic extract of Withania somnifera
fruits decreased fertility in male Wistar rats.

Mahadi and coworkers[26] examined the effect of Withania somnifera
roots (WS) on stress and infertility in men. Normozoospermic fertile men (n=60) not under any stress were assigned to the control
group and normozoospermic infertile men (n=60) were assigned to
the study group, The study group was divided into three subgroups:
i) normozoospermic heavy smokers; ii) normozoospermics under
psychological stress; and iii) normozoospermics with infertility of
unknown etiology. The men in the study group were prescribed WS
(single dose, 5 g/day, P.O) with a cup of skim milk for 3 months.
Several relevant tests were done before and after the study period.
The pregnancy of subjects' partners was noted for 3 months after
the treatment. The following observations were made in the study
group compared to the control group before the treatment:

- lower sperm concentration, slightly lower motility and higher
  semen liquefaction time
- higher LPO and lower SOD, CAT, GSH and ascorbic acid
  in seminal plasma
- lower serum testosterone and LH and higher FSH and PRL
- higher serum cortisol

After the treatment, most of these changes were reduced in all three
subgroups. Three months after the treatment, 14% of subjects' partners achieved pregnancy.

Ahmad and coworkers[27] investigated the effect of Withania somnifera roots (WS) on the semen profile, oxidative biomarkers and
reproductive hormone levels in infertile men. Normal healthy fertile
men (n=75) and infertile men (n=75) were assigned to the control
and study groups respectively. The study group consisted of 3 subgroups: i) normozoospermic infertile men (n=25) who had a normal
(control) semen profile and infertility of unknown etiology; ii) oligozoospermic infertile men (n=25) who had a low sperm count; iii)
asthenozoospermic infertile men (n=25) who had low sperm motility. Subjects in the study group were prescribed WS (5 g/day, P.O.)

with milk for 3 months. Several relevant tests were done before and after the treatment. The following observations were made in the study group compared to the control group before the treatment:

- lower sperm concentration, sperm count per ejaculate and sperm motility
- increased LPO and protein carbonyl groups and decreased SOD, CAT and GSH in seminal plasma
- lower levels of vitamin A, E, C and corrected fructose in seminal plasma
- lower serum levels of LH, T and higher levels of FSH and PRL

Treating infertile men with WS relieved oxidative stress and regulated sex hormone levels.

In a similar investigation, Shukla and coworkers[28] made the following preteatment observations in the study group compared to controls:

- increased intracellular ROS concentration in the spermatozoa and decreased seminal concentration of the metal ions Cu^{2+}, Zn^{2+}, Fe^{2+} and Au^{2+}
- more total (early+late) apoptotic cells in the normozoospermic and oligozoospermic groups
- more late apoptotic and necrotic cells in the asthenozoospermic group

Treating the study group with WS for 3 months caused a decrease in ROS concentration and an increase in metal ion concentration. Also, the number of sperm cells in early and late apoptotic stages diminished. There was no necrosis. The authors concluded that "W. somnifera improves semen quality by reducing oxidative stress and cell death, as well as improving essential metal ion concentrations".

Ambiye and coworkers[29] conducted a study to evaluate the spermatogenic activity of a special extract of Withania somnifera roots (WS) in oligospermic males. 46 male patients with oligospermia were randomly divided into a treatment group (n=21) and a placebo group (n=25). The treatment group received WS (675 mg/day in three doses) for 3 months and the placebo group received a placebo in the same protocol. Semen parameters and serum hormone levels were determined before and after treatment. After completion of the treatment, the treatment group showed a significant increase in sperm concentration, sperm motility, semen volume and serum testosterone compared to baseline. The placebo group showed only small increases compared to baseline. The authors concluded that "The present study adds to the evidence on the therapeutic value of Ashwagandha (Withania somnifera), as attributed in Ayurveda for the treatment of oligospermia leading to infertility".

Dongre and coworkers[30] showed that a special extract of Withania somnifera roots improved sexual function in healthy women.

Mamidi and coworkers[31] examined the efficacy of Withania somnifera in treating psychogenic erectile dysfunction. The results showed that Withania somnifera was no better than placebo in the management of psychogenic erectile dysfunction.

References

1   Maya N. Mascarenhas, Seth R. Flaxman, Ties Boerma, Sheryl Vanderpoel, Gretchen A. Stevens. National, regional, and global trends in infertility prevalence since 1990: a systematic analysis of 277 health surveys. PLOS Medicine (2012) 9 (12): e1001356.

2   P. K. Dalal, Adarsh Tripathi, S. K. Gupta. Vajikarana: Treatment of sexual dysfunction based on Indian concepts. Indian J Psychiatry (2013) 55: 273–276.

3   Shalini R, Jolly Kutty Eapen, Deepa MS. A literature review on Ashwagandha (Withania somnifera (Linn) Dunal): An Ayurvedic aphrodisiac drug. International Ayurvedic Medical Journal (2017) 5(10): 3961-3969.

4   A. A. Al-Qarawi, H. A. Abdel-Rehman, A. A. El-Badry, F. Harraz, N. A. Razig, and E. M. Abdel-Magied. The effect of extracts of Cynomorium coccineum and Withania somnifera on gonadotrophins and ovarian follicles of immature Wistar rats. Phytotherapy Research (2000) 14: 288-290.

5   E. M. Abdel-Magied, H. A. Abdel-Rahman, F. M. Harraz. The effect of aqueous extracts of Cynomorium coccineum and Withania somnifera on testicular development in immature Wistar rats. Journal of Ethnopharmacology (2001) 75: 1-4.

6   Zahra Kiasalari, Mohsen Khalili, Mahbobeh Aghaei. Effect of Withania somnifera on levels of sex hormones in the diabetic male rats. Iranian Journal of Reproductive Medicine (2009) 7(4): 163-168.

7   R Rajashree, M. I. Glad Mohesh, M. V. Ravishankar, Prema Sembulingam. Effect of alcoholic extract of Withania somnifera linn roots on reproductive organs in streptozotocin induced diabetic rats. Indian Journal of Public Health Research & Development (2011) 2 (1): 20-23.

8   Chandrashekara Nagaraj Kyathanahalli, Mallayya Jayawanth Manjunath, Muralidhara. Oral supplementation of standardized extract of Withania somnifera protects against diabetes-induced testicular oxidative impairments in prepubertal rats. Protoplasma (2014) 251 (5): 1021-1029.

9   Nehal M. Belal, Eman M. El-Metwally and Ibrahim S. Salem. Effect of dietary intake Ashwagandha roots powder on the levels of sex hormones in the diabetic and non-diabetic male rats. World Journal of Dairy & Food Sciences (2012) 7 (2): 160-166.

10   Ranjit Kumar, Snehasish Das, Ishita Nanda, Arun Kumar, Md Ali, A. Nath and J. K. Singh. To study bioremedial effect of Withania somnifera on sperm count and seminiferous tubules of endosulfan exposed mice. Global J Trad

Med Sys (2012) 1 (1): 16-20.

11 Ranjit Kumar, Md. Ali, Arun Kumar and Vibha Gahlot. Comparative bioremedial effect of Withania somnifera and Curcuma longa on ovaries of pesticide induced mice. European Journal of Pharmaceutical and Medical Research (2015) 2 (7): 249-253.

12 Nakuleshwar Dut Jasuja, Preeti Sharma and Suresh C. Joshi. Ameliorating effect of Withania somnifera on acephate administered male albino rats. African Journal of Pharmacy and Pharmacology (2013) 7 (23): 1554-1559.

13 Rahul B. Patil, Shreya R. Vora and Meena M. Pillai. Protective effect of spermatogenic activity of Withania somnifera (Ashwagandha) in galactose stressed mice. Annals of Biological Research (2012) 3 (8): 4159-4165.

14 N. H. Shaikh, S. R. Desai and M. V. Walvekar. Protective effects of glycowithanolides on antioxidative enzymes in testes and accessory reproductive organs of D-galactose induced stressed mice. International Journal of Current Microbiology and Applied Sciences (2014) 3 (4): 458-464.

15 Nilofar H Shaikh, Vidya M Deshmukh, Madhuri V Walvekar. Alteration in testicular morphology and sperm count due to glycowithanolides treatment during aging. Asian Journal of Pharmaceutical and Clinical Research (2015) 8(3): 72-77.

16 D. Kaspate, A. R. Ziyaurrahman, T. Saldanha, P. More, S. Toraskar, K. Darak, S. Rohankhedkar and S. Narkhede. To study an aphrodisiac activity of hydroalcoholic extract of Withania somnifera dried roots in female Wistar rats. International Journal of Pharmaceutical Sciences and Research (2015) 6 (7): 2820-2836.

17 Batool Rahmati, Mohammad Hassan Ghosian Moghaddam, Mohsen Khalili, Ehsan Enayati, Maryam Maleki, Saeedeh Rezaeei. Effect of Withania somnifera (L.) Dunal on sex hormones and gonadotropin levels in addicted male rats. International Journal of Fertility and Sterility (2016) 10 (2): 239-244.

18 Arun Kumar, Ranjit Kumar, Mohammad Samuir Rahman, Mohammad Asif Iqubal, Gautam Anand, Pinto Kumar Niraj, Mohammad Ali. Phytoremedial effect of Withania somnifera against arsenic-induced testicular toxicity in Charles Foster rats. Avicenna Journal of Phytomedicine (2015) 5 (4): 355-364.

19 Elumalai Prithiviraj, Sekar Suresh, Nagella Venkata Lakshmi, Mohanraj Karthik Ganesh, Lakshmanan Ganesh, Seppan Prakash. Protective effect of Withania somnifera (Linn.) on cadmium-induced oxidative injury in rat testis. Phytopharmacology (2013) 4 (2): 269-290.

20 S. Saritha, P. Sreenivasulu Reddy, G. Rajarami Reddy. Partial recovery of suppressed reproduction by Withania somnifera Dunal in female rats following perinatal lead exposure. International Journal of Green Pharmacy (2011) 5 (2): 121-125.

21 Divya Bhargavan, B. Deepa, Harish Shetty, A. P. Krishna. The protective effect of Withania somnifera against oxidative damage caused by ethanol in the testes of adult male rats, International Journal of Basic & Clinical Pharmacology (2015) 4 (6): 1104-1108.

22 Divyashree S and Yajurvedi H N. Efficacy of the herb Withania somnifera L in the prevention of stress-induced alterations in the ovary of rat. International Journal of Pharma and Bio Sciences (2017) 8 (1): 283-290.

23 I. Ilayperuma, W. D. Ratnasooriya, T. R. Weerasooriya. Effect of Withania somnifera root extract on the sexual behavior of male rats. Asian Journal of Andrology (2002) 4(4): 295-298.

24 Ashish Ranjan Singh, Kapil Singh, Preetam Singh Shekhawat. Spermicidal activity and antifertility activity of ethanolic extract of Withania somnifera in

male albino rats. International Journal of Pharmaceutical Sciences Review and Research (2013) 21 (2): 227-232.

25 Pratap Chand Mali. Control of fertility in male Wistar rats treated with hydroalcoholic extract of Withania somnifera fruits. International Journal of Pharmacology & Biological sciences (2013) 7 (3): 14-21.

26 Abbas Ali Mahdi, Kamla Kant Shukla, Mohammad Kaleem Ahmad, Singh Rajender, Satya Narain Shankhwar, Vishwajeet Singh and Deepansh Dalela. Withania somnifera improves semen quality in stress-related male fertility. eCAM 2009. doi: 10.1093/ecam/nep138

27 Mohammad Kaleem Ahmad, Abbas Ali Mahdi, Kamla Kant Shukla, Najmul Islam, Singh Rajender, Dama Madhukar, Satya Narain Shankhwar and Sohail Ahmad. Withania somnifera improves semen quality by regulating reproductive hormone levels and oxidative stress in seminal plasma of infertile males. Fertility and Sterility (2010) 94 (3): 989-996.

28 Kamla Kant Shukla, Abbas Ali Mahdi, Vivek Mishra, Singh Rajender, Satya Narain Sankhwar, Devender Patel, Mukul Das. Withania somnifera improves semen quality by combating oxidative stress and cell death and improving essential metal concentrations. Reproductive Biomedicine Online (2011) 22: 421-427.

29 Vijay R. Ambiye, Deepak Langade, Swati Dongre, Pradnya Aptikar, Madhura Kulkarni, and Atul Dongre. Clinical evaluation of the spermatogenic activity of the root of Ashwagandha (Withania somnifera) in oligospermic males: A pilot study. Evidence-Based Complementary and Alternative Medicine, vol. 2013, Article ID571420.

30 Swati Dongre, Deepak Langade, and Sauvik Bhattacharya. Efficacy and safety of Ashwagandha (Withania somnifera) root extract in improving sexual function in women: A pilot study. Biomed Research International, vol. 2015, Article ID 284154.

31 Prasad Mamidi, Kshama Gupta, Anup B Thakar. Ashwagandha in psychogenic erectile dysfunction: Ancillary findings. Int. J. Res. Ayurveda Pharm (2014) 5 (1): 36-40.

20 – Safety-related Issues and Conclusion

20.1 – Introduction

Withania somnifera has been extensively used for a long time by Ayurvedic practitioners to treat a variety of ailments. It has been included in the GRAS (generally recognized as safe) family of herbal plants based on toxicological studies[1]. However, systematic human studies on the safety and efficacy of Withania somnifera are lacking. Results from some toxicological studies and safety-related issues are summarized below.

20.2 – Toxicity Studies

Singh and coworkers[2] determined the LD_{50} value in mice of an alcoholic extract of Withania somnifera defatted seeds. In acute toxicity studies with albino mice, LD_{50} (P.O.) was 1750 mg/kg.

Ghosal and coworkers[3] examined the acute toxicity in mice of sitoindosides IX and X isolated from Withania somnifera. Swiss albino mice were treated with sitoindoside IX or X (100-1000 mg/kg, P.O. or i.p). No mortality was observed in mice treated orally with sitoindoside IX or X for 24 hours. The intraperitoneal LD_{50} values of sitoindosides IX and X were 518 mg/kg and 808 mg/kg respectively.

Malhotra and coworkers[4] tested the toxicity of ashwagandholine (total alkaloids from Withania somnifera roots) in rats and mice. A suspension of ashwagandholine (2%) was prepared in 10% glycol using 2% gum acacia as a suspending agent. The acute LD_{50} for this preparation was 465 mg/kg (332-651 mg/kg) in rats and 432 mg/kg (299-626 mg/kg) in mice.

Sharada and coworkers[5] examined the toxicity of a Withania somnifera root extract (WSR) in rats and mice. In the acute toxicity study (24 h), Swiss albino mice were treated with WSR (1100-1500 mg/kg, i.p.). No mortality was observed at 1100 mg/kg and LD_{50} was 1260 mg/kg. In the subacute toxicity study, Wistar rats were injected with WSR (100 mg/kg/day) for 30 days. No mortality or changes in peripheral blood constituents were observed. However, a significant decrease in the weight of the spleen and adrenals was observed in male rats. Another investigation[6] evaluated the acute toxicity of Withaferin A (WA) in mice. Overnight fasted albino mice were treated with WA (30-140 mg/kg, i.p.) and monitored for 14 days. No mortality was observed at the 30 or 40 mg/kg doses. Mortality was marginal up to 60 mg/kg and increased sharply above 70 mg/kg. LD_{50} was 80 mg/kg.

Prabhu and coworkers[7] investigated the toxicity of a hydroalcoholic extract of Withania somnifera roots (WSR) in rats. In the acute study, rats were treated with WSR (2000 mg/kg, P.O.) and monitored for 14 days. No signs of toxicity or mortality were observed. In the subacute study, rats were treated with WSR (500, 1000 or 2000 mg/kg/day, P.O.) for 28 days. No signs of toxicity or mortality were observed. No significant changes were observed in body weight, organ weight, hematological parameters or biochemical parameters. No gross/histopathological lesions were observed. Another study[8] evaluated the prenatal developmental toxicity of a Withania somnifera root extract (WSR) in Wistar rats. Pregnant rats were treated with WSR (500, 1000 or 2000 mg/kg, P.O.) during the period of major organogenesis and histogenesis (gestation days 5-19). No evidence of maternal or fetal toxicity was observed. The treatment did not cause significant changes in the body weight of parental females or in the number of corpora lutea, implantations, viable fetuses or external, skeletal and visceral malformations.

Patel and coworkers[9] evaluated the toxicity of a Withania somnifera extract (WSE) in Wistar rats. In the acute study, rats were treated with WSE (2000 mg/kg, P.O.) and monitored for 14 days. No toxic effects were observed and LD_{50} was estimated to be greater than 2000 mg/kg. In the subacute study, rats were treated with WSE (500, 1000 or 2000 mg/kg, via oral gavage) for 28 days. No treatment-related adverse effects were observed.

In an acute toxicity study, Mukhopadhyay and coworkers[10] observed no mortality or behavioral changes in adult Swiss albino mice treated with a proprietary formulation containing a Withania somnifera root extract (up to 2000 mg/kg) after 14 days of treatment.

Hussein and coworkers[11] examined the toxicity of an alcoholic extract of Withania somnifera aerial parts (leaves, stems, and fruits) in rats. In the acute study (24 h), rats were treated (i.p.) with 150-1200 mg/kg of the extract. LD_{50} was 522 mg/kg. In the subchronic study, rats were treated (i.p.) with 52, 104 or 208 mg/kg 4 times a week for 60 days. Rats treated with 104 and 208 mg of the extract showed 15% and 20% mortality respectively.

Antony and coworkers[12] evaluated the toxicity of a purified Ashwagandha extract (PAE) in rats. The extract contained 35% glycowithanolides and less than 1% alkaloids. In the acute study, female rats were treated with PAE (2000 mg/kg, P.O.). No signs of toxicity or mortality were observed after 14 days. The estimated LD_{50} value was greater than 2000 mg/kg. In the subchronic toxicity study, rats were treated with PAE (1000 mg/kg/day, P.O.) for 90 days. No signs of toxicity or mortality were observed. No significant difference between the hematology or biochemistry profiles of PAE-treated rats and controls was observed. The histopathology of major organs in the PAE-treated group was similar to the control group.

Bhattacharya and coworkers[13] examined the acute toxicity in mice of a methanol-water (1:1) extract of Withania somnifera roots (SG-1) and an equimolar combination of sitoindosides VII, VIII and Withaferin A (SG-2). The intraperitoneal LD_{50} values of SG-1 and SG-2 were 1076 mg/kg and 1564 mg/kg respectively.

Raut and coworkers[14] conducted an exploratory study to evaluate the tolerability, safety and activity of Ashwagandha in healthy subjects. Healthy subjects (12 males and 6 females, all volunteers) were selected for the study. Gelatine capsules containing a Withania somnifera extract (250, 500 or 750 mg/capsule) were used. On days 1-10, each subject received one 250 mg capsule in the morning and one 500 mg capsule at night. On days 11-20, each subject received one 500 mg capsule in the morning and one 500 mg capsule at night. On days 21-30, each subject received one 500 mg capsule in the morning and one 750 mg capsule at night. All subjects except for one experienced beneficial effects. One subject who reported an unusual increase in appetite, libido and hallucinogenic effects with vertigo was withdrawn from the study on the 6th day and the symptoms disappeared within a couple of days.

Chandrasekhar and coworkers[15] demonstrated the safety and efficacy of a full-spectrum extract of Ashwagandha roots in reducing stress and anxiety in adults. In this study, 64 subjects complaining of mental stress were divided randomly into a placebo (n=32) group and drug study (n=32) group. Each subject in the drug study group received one Ashwagandha capsule (300 mg/capsule) two times a day after food for 60 days. The subjects in the placebo group received placebo capsules. After the treatment, subjects in the drug study group showed a significant improvement in handling stress compared to the placebo group. No major adverse effects were reported.

20.3 – Herb-Drug Interactions

Care must be exercised while taking Withania somnifera along with drugs used to treat diabetes, hypertension, anxiety, depression, immunological disorders and thyroid disorders.

20.4 – Adverse Side Effects

Withania somnifera is generally well tolerated. However, transient minor side effects such as diarrhea, vomiting and abdominal pain have been reported. Pregnant and breastfeeding women are advised to avoid Withania somnifera.

20.5 – Conclusion

The available scientific data from a large number of in vitro and in vivo investigations as well as a limited number of human clinical trials indicate multiple areas of therapeutic potential for Withania somnifera. It seems that Withania somnifera has positive effects on the endocrine, cardiopulmonary and central nervous systems. However, large scale human trials with standardized formulations of Withania somnifera are needed to provide a strong scientific basis for medicinal applications. As with other herbal products, areas of concern include contamination by pesticides, herbicides, heavy metals, toxins and adulteration by other means.

References

1   B. Jayaprakasam, Y. Zhang, N. P. Seeram, M.G. Nair. Growth inhibition of tumor cell lines by Withanolides from Withania somnifera leaves. Life Sci (2003) 74 (1): 125-132.
2   N. Singh, R. Nath, A. Lata, S. P. Singh, R. P. Kohli and K. P. Bhargava. Withania somnifera (Ashwagandha), a rejuvenating herbal drug which enhances survival during stress (an adaptogen). Int. J. Crude Drug Res (1982) 20 (1): 29-35.
3   Shibanath Ghosal, Jawahar Lal, Radheyshyam Srivastava, Salil K. Bhattacharya, Sachidananda N. Upadhyay, Arun K. Jaiswal, Uptala Chattopadhyay. Immunomodulatory and CNS effects of sitoindosides IX and X, two new glycowithanolides from Withania somnifera. Phytotherapy Research (1989) 3 (5): 201-206.
4   C. L. Malhotra, V. L. Mehta, P. K. Das and N. S. Dhalla. Studies on Withania-Ashwagandha, Kaul (part-V): The effect of total alkaloids (ashwagandholine) on the central nervous system. Indian J Physiol Pharmacol (1965) 9 (3): 127-36.
5   A. C. Sharada, F. Emerson Solomon & P. Uma Devi. Toxicity of Withania somnifera root extract in rats and mice. International Journal of Pharmacognosy (1993) 31 (3): 205-212.

6   A. Chandrashekar Sharada, F. Emerson Solomon, Pathirisseri Uma Devi, Nayanabhirama Udupa. & K. Kaitheri Srinivasan. Antitumor and radiosensitizing effects of Withaferin A on mouse Ehrlich ascites carcinoma in vivo. Acta Oncologica (1996) 35 (1): 95-100.

7   P. C. Prabu, S. Panchapakesan, C. David Raj. Acute and sub-acute oral toxicity assessment of the hydroalcoholic extract of Withania somnifera roots in Wistar rats. Phytotherapy Research (2013) 27 (8): 1169-1178.

8   P. C. Prabu & S. Panchapakesan. Prenatal developmental toxicity evaluation of Withania somnifera root extract I Wistar rats. Drug and Chemical Toxicology (2015) 38 (1): 50-56.

9   Shruti B. Patel, Nirav J. Rao, Lal L. Hingorani. Safety assessment of Withania somnifera extract standardized for Withaferin A: acute and sub-acute toxicity study. Journal of Ayurveda and Integrative Medicine (2016) 7: 30-37.

10 Anindya Mukhopadhyay, Raja Chakraverty, Himangshu Sekhar Maji. Evaluation of the safety and efficacy of an Ayurvedic proprietary medicine containing roots of Withania somnifera. Indo American Journal of Pharmaceutical Research (2016) 6 (8).

11 Yehia A. Hussein, Saad S. Al-Shokair, Khaled M. Ashry. Acute and sub-chronic toxicological potential of Withania somnifera extract on rats. Alexandria Journal of Veterinary Sciences (2017) 55 (2): 10-18.

12 Benny Antony, Merina Benny, Binu T Kuruvilla, Nishant Kumar Gupta, Anu Sebastian, Sherina Jacob. Acute and sub chronic studies of purified Withania somnifera extract in rats. International Journal of Pharmacy and Pharmaceutical Sciences (2018) 10 (12): 41-46.

13 Salil K. Bhattacharya, Raj K. Goel, Ravinder Kaur and Shibnath Ghosal. Anti-stress activity of sitoindosides VII and VIII, new acylsterylglucosides from Withania somnifera. Phytotherapy Research (1987) 1(1): 32-37.

14 Ashwinikumar A. Raut, Nirmala N. Rege, Firoz M. Tadvi, Punita V. Solanki, Kirti R. Kene, Sudatta G. Shirolkar, Shefali N. Pandey, Rama A. Vaidya, Ashok B. Vaidya. Exploratory study to evaluate tolerability and activity of Ashwagandha (Withania somnifera) in healthy volunteers. Journal of Ayurveda and Integrative Medicine (2012) 3 (3): 111-114.

15 K. Chandrasekhar, Jyoti Kapoor, and Sridhar Anishetty. A prospective, randomized double-blind, placebo-controlled study of safety and efficacy of a high-concentration full-spectrum extract of Ashwagandha root in reducing stress and anxiety in adults. Indian Journal of Psychological Medicine (2012) 34 (3): 252-262.

Common Abbreviations

AChE – acetylcholinesterase

ACTH – adenocorticotropic hormone

Akt, PKB – protein kinase B

ALP – alkaline phosphate

ALT, ALAT, SGPT – alanine aminotransferase

AMPA – α-amino-3-hydroxy-5-methyl-4-isoxazolepropionic acid

AST, ASAT, SGOT – aspartate aminotransferase

AP-1 – activator protein-1

BChE – butyrylcholinesterase

BHA – butylated hydroxyanisole

BHT – butylated hydroxytoluene

BUN – blood urea nitrogen

CAT – catalase

ChAT – choline acetyltransferase

CMC – carboxymethyl cellulose

Con A – concanavalin A

COX-2 – cyclooxygenase-2

CPK – creatine phosphokinase

CRP – C-reactive protein

DA – dopamine

DHAES – dehydroepiandrosterone sulfate

DOPAC – 3,4-dihydroxyphenylacetic acid

DR – death receptor

EDTA – ethylenediaminetetraacetic acid

EMT – epithelial to mesenchymal transition

ER – estrogen

ERK – extracellular signal-regulated kinase

FSH – follicle stimulating hormone

GAD – glutamate decarboxylase

GGT – gamma-glutamyltransferase

GLAST – glutamate aspartate transporter

GM-CSF – granulocyte-macrophage colony-stimulating factor

GPx, GSHPx – glutathione peroxidase

G6PDH – glucose-6-phosphate dehydrogenase

GR, GRx – glutathione reductase

GSH – reduced glutathione

GSSH – oxidized glutathione

GST – glutathione S-transferase

HbA1c – hemoglobin A1c

HO-1 – heme oxygenase-1

HER-2 – human epidermal growth factor receptor 2

H_2O_2 – hydrogen peroxide

HP – hydroperoxide

3β-HSD – 3-beta-hydroxysteroid dehydrogenase

HVA – homovanillic acid

IFN-γ – interferon gamma

iNOS – inducible nitric oxide synthase

IKK – inhibitor of kappa kinase

IP3 – inositol triphosphate

JAK – janus kinase

α-KGDH – alpha-ketoglutarate dehydrogenase

LDH – lactate dehydrogenase

LDL-C – low-density lipoprotein cholesterol

HDL-C – high-density lipoprotein cholesterol

VLDL-C – very low-density lipoprotein cholesterol

LPS – lipopolysaccharide

MAPK – mitogen-activated protein kinase

Mad-Cdc – mitotic arrest deficient-cell division cycle

MDA – malondialdehyde

MDH – malate dehydrogenase

NADPH – reduced nicotinamide adenine dinucleotide phosphate

NF-κB – nuclear factor kappa B

NIDDM – non-insulin dependent diabetes mellitus

NMDA – N-methyl-D-aspartate

PARP – poly (ADP-ribose) polymerase

PAR-4 – prostate apoptosis response-4

PC – protein carbonyl

PR – progesterone

RET – rearranged during transfection

RSK – ribosomal S6 kinase

SDH – succinate dehydrogenase

SOD – superoxide dismutase

SRBC – sheep red blood cells

STAT3 – signal transducer and activator of transcription 3

T – testosterone

T3 – triiodothyronine

T4 – thyroxine

TSH – thyroid stimulating hormone

TBARS – thiobarbituric acid derivatives

TC – total cholesterol

TG – triglycerides

TGF – transforming growth factor

TNF – tumor necrosis factor

TH – reduced tyrosine hydroxylase

VEGF – vascular endothelial growth factor